T0361829

Updates on Osteoporosis

Editor

PAULINE M. CAMACHO

ENDOCRINOLOGY AND METABOLISM CLINICS OF NORTH AMERICA

www.endo.theclinics.com

Consulting Editor
ADRIANA G. IOACHIMESCU

June 2021 • Volume 50 • Number 2

ELSEVIER

1600 John F. Kennedy Boulevard • Suite 1800 • Philadelphia, Pennsylvania, 19103-2899

http://www.theclinics.com

**ENDOCRINOLOGY AND METABOLISM CLINICS OF NORTH AMERICA Volume 50, Number 2
June 2021 ISSN 0889-8529, ISBN 13: 978-0-323-79551-7**

Editor: Katerina Heidhausen
Developmental Editor: Jessica Cañaberal

Endocrinology and Metabolism Clinics of North America (ISSN 0889-8529) is published quarterly by Elsevier Inc., 360 Park Avenue South, New York, NY 10010-1710. Months of issue are March, June, September, and December. Periodicals postage paid at New York, NY and additional mailing offices. Subscription prices are USD 383.00 per year for US individuals, USD 1037.00 per year for US institutions, USD 100.00 per year for US students and residents, USD 454.00 per year for Canadian individuals, USD 1089.00 per year for Canadian institutions, USD 497.00 per year for international individuals, USD 1089.00 per year for international institutions, USD 100.00 per year for Canadian students/residents, and USD 245.00 per year for international students/residents. To receive student/resident rate, orders must be accompanied by name of affiliated institution, date of term, and the signature of program/residency coordinator on institution letterhead. Orders will be billed at individual rate until proof of status is received. Foreign air speed delivery is included in all *Clinics* subscription prices. All prices are subject to change without notice. **POSTMASTER:** Send address changes to *Endocrinology and Metabolism Clinics of North America*, Elsevier Health Sciences Division, Subscription Customer Service, 3251 Riverport Lane, Maryland Heights, MO 63043. **Customer Service: Telephone: 1-800-654-2452** (U.S. and Canada); **1-314-447-8871** (outside U.S. and Canada). **Fax: 1-314-447-8029. E-mail: journalscustomerservice-usa@elsevier.com (for print support); journalsonlinesupport-usa@elsevier.com (for online support)**.

Reprints. For copies of 100 or more, of articles in this publication, please contact the Commercial Rights Department, Elsevier Inc., 360 Park Avenue South, New York, NY 10010-1710; phone: +1-212-633-3874; fax: +1-212-633-3820; E-mail: reprints@elsevier.com.

Endocrinology and Metabolism Clinics of North America is covered in *MEDLINE/PubMed (Index Medicus)*, *EMBASE/Excerpta Medica, Current Contents/Clinical Medicine, Current Contents/Life Sciences, Science Citation Index, ISI/BIOMED, BIOSIS,* and *Chemical Abstracts*.

Contributors

CONSULTING EDITOR

ADRIANA G. IOACHIMESCU, MD, PhD, FACE
Professor, Departments of Medicine, Endocrinology and Metabolism, and Neurosurgery, Emory University, Emory University School of Medicine, Atlanta, Georgia, USA

EDITOR

PAULINE M. CAMACHO, MD, FACE
Professor of Medicine, Division of Endocrinology and Metabolism, Loyola University Medical Center, Director, Loyola Osteoporosis and Metabolic Bone Disease Center, Maywood, Illinois, USA

AUTHORS

ROBERT A. ADLER, MD
Chief, Endocrinology and Metabolism, Central Virginia Veterans Affairs Health Care System, Professor of Internal Medicine, Division of Endocrinology, Virginia Commonwealth University, Richmond, Virginia, USA

ROD MARIANNE ARCEO-MENDOZA, MD
Assistant Professor, Department of Endocrinology, Loyola Osteoporosis and Metabolic Bone Disease Center, Loyola University Medical Center, Maywood, Illinois, USA

PAULINE M. CAMACHO, MD, FACE
Professor of Medicine, Division of Endocrinology and Metabolism, Loyola University Medical Center, Director, Loyola Osteoporosis and Metabolic Bone Disease Center, Maywood, Illinois, USA

BART L. CLARKE, MD
Professor of Medicine, Mayo Clinic, Rochester, Minnesota, USA

DIMA L. DIAB, MD, FACE, FACP, CCD
Associate Professor of Clinical Medicine, Division of Endocrinology/Metabolism, Department of Internal Medicine, Cincinnati VA Medical Center, University of Cincinnati Bone Health and Osteoporosis, Cincinnati, Ohio, USA

LAURA T. DICKENS, MD
Section of Adult and Pediatric Endocrinology, Diabetes, and Metabolism, Department of Medicine, University of Chicago, Chicago, Illinois, USA

MATTHEW T. DRAKE, MD, PhD
Division of Endocrinology, Diabetes, Metabolism and Nutrition, Robert and Arlene Kogod Center on Aging, Mayo Clinic, Rochester, Minnesota, USA

SUMEET JAIN, MD
Assistant Professor, Department of Medicine, Division of Endocrinology and Metabolism, Rush University Medical Center, Chicago, Illinois, USA

WILLIAM D. LESLIE, MD, FRCPC, MSc
Department of Medicine, Rady Faculty of Health Sciences, University of Manitoba, Winnipeg, Manitoba, Canada

E. MICHAEL LEWIECKI, MD
Clinical Assistant Professor of Medicine, University of New Mexico Health Sciences Center, Director, Bone Health TeleECHO, Director, New Mexico Clinical Research and Osteoporosis Center, Albuquerque, New Mexico, USA

SANDRA C. NAAMAN, MD, PhD
Section of General Internal Medicine, Department of Medicine, University of Chicago, Chicago, Illinois, USA

DOMINIK SAUL, MD
Division of Endocrinology, Diabetes, Metabolism and Nutrition, Robert and Arlene Kogod Center on Aging, Mayo Clinic, Rochester, Minnesota, USA; Department of Trauma Surgery, Orthopaedics and Plastic Surgery, University of Göttingen, Göttingen, Germany

G. ISANNE SCHACTER, MD, FRCPC
Department of Medicine, Rady Faculty of Health Sciences, University of Manitoba, Winnipeg, Manitoba, Canada

NELSON B. WATTS, MD, FACP, MACE, CCD
Director, Mercy Health Osteoporosis and Bone Health Services, Cincinnati, Ohio, USA

GUIDO ZAVATTA, MD
Mayo Clinic, Rochester, Minnesota, USA; Division of Endocrinology and Diabetes Prevention and Care, IRCCS Azienda Ospedaliero-Universitaria di Bologna, Department of Medical and Surgical Sciences (DIMEC), Alma Mater Studiorum, University of Bologna, Bologna, Italy

MELTEM ZEYTINOGLU, MD, MBA
Section of Adult and Pediatric Endocrinology, Diabetes, and Metabolism, Department of Medicine, University of Chicago, Chicago, Illinois, USA

Contents

> Significant development has occurred in the treatment of postmenopausal osteoporosis. We review the most recent guidelines from the American Association of Clinical Endocrinologists/American College of Endocrinology, Endocrine Society, and the European Society for Clinical and Economic Aspects of Osteoporosis and Osteoarthritis/International Osteoporosis Foundation Guidelines.

> Osteoporosis is characterized by reduced bone mass leading to diminished skeletal integrity and an increased risk for fracture. Multiple agents exist that are effective for the treatment of osteoporosis. These can be broadly categorized into those that reduce the risk for additional loss of bone mass (anti-resorptive agents) and those that augment existing bone mass (anabolic agents). This article reviews the different medications within each class, and discusses more recent data regarding the combination and sequential use of these medications for optimization of skeletal health in patients at high risk for fracture.

> Bisphosphonates remain a first-line treatment for osteoporosis and decrease vertebral and hip fractures without side effects in most patients. With extended treatment, osteonecrosis of the jaw and atypical femoral fracture occur rarely, but fear of side effects has led to not starting or discontinuing treatment. Atrial fibrillation and uveitis are less appreciated by the general public, but their rare incidence must be recognized. A strategy for safe long-term treatment is provided based on 2 major studies. Interruption of treatment after 3 to 5 years is possible for some patients, but those remaining at high fracture risk require longer term therapy.

Both diabetes and osteoporosis are increasingly prevalent diseases, in part owing to aging populations worldwide. Epidemiologic data have shown that other organs may be adversely affected by diabetes, including the skeleton, in what has become known as diabetes-induced osteoporosis, which represents the combined impact of conventional osteoporosis with the additional fracture burden attributed to diabetes. There is an increased risk of fracture in patients with Type 1 and Type 2 diabetes, and some antidiabetic medications also may contribute to increased risk of fracture in diabetes.

Diabetes-induced osteoporosis is characterized by an increase in fracture risk. FRAX, the most widely used tool, underestimates the risk of fracture in both type 1 and type 2 diabetes. Specific adjustments to FRAX can help to better identify patients with diabetes at increased risk of fracture and select those at high fracture risk for treatment. Although clinical trial data are limited, the available evidence indicates that the presence of diabetes does not alter antiosteoporotic treatment response in patients with diabetes.

A bone fractures when a force applied to it exceeds its strength. Assessment of bone strength is an important component in determining the risk of fracture and guiding treatment decisions. Dual-energy X-ray absorptiometry is used to diagnosis osteoporosis, estimate fracture risk, and monitor changes in bone density. Fracture risk algorithms provide enhanced fracture risk predictability. Advanced technologies with computed tomography (CT) and MRI can measure parameters of bone microarchitecture. Mathematical modeling using CT data can evaluate the behavior of bone structures in response to external loading. Microindentation techniques directly measure the strength of outer bone cortex.

ENDOCRINOLOGY AND METABOLISM CLINICS OF NORTH AMERICA

SERIES OF RELATED INTEREST

Medical Clinics
https://www.medical.theclinics.com
Primary Care: Clinics in Office Practice
https://www.primarycare.theclinics.com/

VISIT THE CLINICS ONLINE!
Access your subscription at:
www.theclinics.com

Foreword
Updates on Osteoporosis

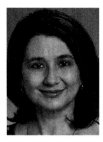

Adriana G. Ioachimescu, MD, PhD, FACE
Consulting Editor

The "Updates on Osteoporosis" issue of the *Endocrinology and Metabolism Clinics of North America* reflects the significant recent progress in management of this highly prevalent condition. The guest editor is Dr Pauline M. Camacho, MD, FACE, Professor of Medicine at Loyola University Medical Center, and Director of the Loyola Osteoporosis and Metabolic Bone Disease Center. Dr Camacho is the first author of the 2020 update to the American Association of Clinical Endocrinologists (AACE)/American College of Endocrinology guidelines on diagnosis and treatment of postmenopausal osteoporosis.

In 2019 and 2020, several societies updated their guidelines for management of postmenopausal osteoporosis, including AACE, the Endocrine Society, and the European Society for Clinical and Economic Aspects of Osteoporosis and Osteoarthritis/International Osteoporosis Foundation. The authors review carefully specific recommendations and emphasize fracture risk stratification, therapy, duration of treatment, and long-term surveillance. While fewer men are affected by osteoporosis than women, the mortality associated with major fragility fractures is higher in men. The authors elaborate on bone densitometry limitations in identifying men at risk for fractures, the importance of evaluation for secondary causes, and treatment choices.

Among conditions associated with secondary osteoporosis, chronic glucocorticoid administration and organ transplantation pose specific management problems, which are thoroughly addressed from pathogenesis to management. In addition, in recent years, the connection between diabetes type 1 and 2 and osteoporosis has emerged; the authors present the most recent knowledge regarding epidemiology, pathogenesis, and impact of antidiabetes medication on fracture risk.

Several classes of medications are available for treatment of osteoporosis, including antiresorptive therapies (bisphosphonates, denosumab, selective estrogen agonists/ antagonists), anabolic agents (teriparatide, abaloparatide), and, more recently,

Endocrinol Metab Clin N Am 50 (2021) ix–x
https://doi.org/10.1016/j.ecl.2021.03.012
0889-8529/21/© 2021 Published by Elsevier Inc.

endo.theclinics.com

antisclerostin monoclonal antibodies (romosozumab). The authors provide important updates on their mechanism of action, adverse effects, drug holidays, and steps toward discontinuation.

Recent data regarding clinical applicability of bone turnover markers in diagnosis and monitoring of osteoporosis treatment are presented along with pitfalls in interpretation. Dual-energy X-ray absorptiometry is the most commonly used technology to measure the bone mineral density and assess fracture risk. The authors examine fracture risk algorithms and advances in bone strength assessment.

I hope you will find this issue of the *Endocrinology and Metabolism Clinics of North America* a great resource for your practice. I would like to thank our guest editor, the authors, and the Elsevier editorial staff for their important contributions.

Adriana G. Ioachimescu, MD, PhD, FACE
Emory University School of Medicine
1365 B Clifton Road, Northeast, B6209
Atlanta, GA 30322, USA

E-mail address:
aioachi@emory.edu

Preface

2021 Updates on Osteoporosis Diagnosis and Therapy

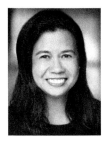

Pauline M. Camacho, MD, FACE
Editor

In this Special Edition of *Endocrinology and Metabolism Clinics of North America*, our objective was to focus on the latest updates on the diagnosis and management of osteoporosis from the past decade. Significant progress has been made in the therapeutics of osteoporosis, with the addition of a new agent and significantly longer clinical experience with established agents. As we have gained knowledge about the therapeutic options, many more questions have arisen. What are the latest guidelines on postmenopausal osteoporosis treatment, and how are they similar or different? What is the ideal initial agent based on patients' fracture risk? How do we use drugs sequentially? When can drugs be discontinued, and what is the safest way to do this? What is the latest information on rare adverse events from osteoporosis agents? In addition, we also present new developments on male, glucocorticoid, and transplant osteoporosis, as well as the impact of diabetes on bone. Finally, we review technological advances in assessing bone quality and bone mass.

On behalf of the authors, I am delighted to present this update on osteoporosis, and I hope that the readers will find this useful in their clinical practice.

Pauline M. Camacho, MD, FACE
Division of Endocrinology and Metabolism
Loyola University Medical Center
Loyola Osteoporosis and
Metabolic Bone Disease Center
2160 South First Avenue, Suite 137
Maywood, IL 60153, USA

E-mail address:
pcamach@lumc.edu

Endocrinol Metab Clin N Am 50 (2021) xi
https://doi.org/10.1016/j.ecl.2021.03.011
0889-8529/21/© 2021 Published by Elsevier Inc.

Postmenopausal Osteoporosis: Latest Guidelines

Rod Marianne Arceo-Mendoza, MD*, Pauline M. Camacho, MD

KEYWORDS

- Postmenopausal osteoporosis • Osteopenia • Fragility fracture • DXA • FRAX
- Treatment guidelines • AACE • ACE

KEY POINTS

- Significant development has occurred in the treatment of Postmenopausal Osteoporosis. We review the most recent guidelines from American Association of Clinical Endocrinologists/American College of Endocrinology (AACE/ACE), Endocrine Society (ES), and European Society for Clinical and Economic Aspects of Osteoporosis and Osteoarthritis/International Osteoporosis Foundation (ESCEO/IOF).
- The new anabolic agent, Romosozumab, is now approved for use in treatment of postmenopausal osteoporosis and is now included in the treatment algorithm in major endocrinology/osteoporosis society guidelines.
- AACE/ACE, ES, and ESCEO/IOF Clinical guidelines highlights the importance of fracture risk assessment to help stratify patients and guide decision-making in pharmacologic therapy.

OSTEOPOROSIS

Osteoporosis is a disease characterized by increased bone turnover and decreased bone mass with associated skeletal fragility, resulting in an increased risk of fracture.[1] It is a well-defined and growing public health problem. The National Osteoporosis Foundation estimates that 10.2 million Americans have osteoporosis and that an additional 43.4 million have low bone mass. It is estimated that by 2030, the number of adults with osteoporosis and low bone mass will increase to 71 million.[2]

More than 2 million osteoporosis-related fractures occur annually in the United States. Approximately 1 in 2 White women and 1 in 5 men will experience an osteoporotic-related fracture in their lifetime. By 2025, the burden in the country is projected to increase by almost 50% to more than 3 million fractures and US$253 billion per year.[3]

Department of Endocrinology, Osteoporosis and Metabolic Bone Disease Center, Loyola University Medical Center, 2160 South 1st Avenue, Maywood, IL 60153, USA
* Corresponding author.
E-mail address: Rmmendoza@lumc.edu

Endocrinol Metab Clin N Am 50 (2021) 167–178
https://doi.org/10.1016/j.ecl.2021.03.009
0889-8529/21/© 2021 Elsevier Inc. All rights reserved.

In 1994, a Working Group of the World Health Organization established an operational definition of osteoporosis based on bone mineral density (BMD). Osteoporosis is defined as a BMD 2.5 SD or more below the average value for premenopausal women.[4] Normal BMD is defined as T-score of −1.0 or higher and a T-score between −1.0 and −2.5 is defined as osteopenia or low bone mass.

Although osteoporosis has traditionally been diagnosed based on low bone density in the absence of fracture, the 2016 and 2020 American Association of Clinical Endocrinologists (AACE)/American College of Endocrinology (ACE) Clinical Practice Guidelines for Diagnosis and Treatment of Postmenopausal Osteoporosis[5] agree that osteoporosis may also be diagnosed in patients with osteopenia and increased fracture risk using FRAX country-specific thresholds (**Table 1**).

DIAGNOSIS

History and physical examination should include assessment of risk factors for fractures as well as secondary causes of osteoporosis (**Box 1**).

The fracture risk assessment tool known as FRAX, introduced in 2008, is a computer-based algorithm (http://www.shef.ac.uk/FRAX) that calculates the 10-year probability of a major osteoporotic fracture (hip, clinical spine, humerus, or wrist fracture) and the 10-year probability of hip fracture.[6] Fracture risk is calculated from age, body mass index, and well-validated dichotomized risk factors (**Table 2**).

The risk factors included in FRAX are listed in **Table 2**. When using the FRAX tool, pharmacologic intervention is recommended for patients with greater than or equal to 20% probability of major osteoporotic fracture or greater than or equal to 3% probability of hip fracture in the next 10 years in the United States, and this may be slightly different in other countries.

TREATMENT
Nonpharmacologic Management

Screening for causes of secondary osteoporosis should be completed and corrected. Preventive therapy, with calcium and vitamin D supplements, and medication compliance and fall prevention need to be stressed to the patients at every visit.

Table 1 Diagnostic criteria		
WHO Criteria for Classification of Osteopenia and Osteoporosis		**2016 and 2020 AACE Diagnosis of Osteoporosis in Postmenopausal Women**
Category	T-score	1. T-score −2.5 or below in the lumbar spine, femoral neck, total proximal femur, or 1/3 radius
Normal	−1.0 or above	
Low bone mass (osteopenia)	Between −1.0 and −2.5	
	−2.5 or below	2. Low-trauma spine or hip fracture (regardless of BMD)
Osteoporosis	−2.5 or below with fragility fracture	3. T-score between −1.0 and −2.5 and a fragility fracture of proximal humerus, pelvis, or distal forearm
Severe or established osteoporosis		4. T-score between −1.0 and −2.5 and high FRAX (or if available, TBS-adjusted FRAX) fracture probability based on country-specific thresholds

Abbreviations: AACE, American Association of Clinical Endocrinologists; BMD, bone mineral density; TBS, trabecular bone score; WHO, World Health Organization.

Box 1
Causes of secondary osteoporosis

Endocrine or Metabolic Causes
  Hyperparathyroidism
  Hypophosphatasia
  Hypercortisolism
  Diabetes
  Adrenal insufficiency
  Hypogonadism
  Hyperthyroidism
  Growth hormone deficiency
  Acromegaly
  Pregnancy

Nutritional and gastrointestinal conditions
  Vitamin D deficiency
  Calcium deficiency
  High caffeine intake
  Anorexia nervosa
  Alcoholism
  Chronic liver disease
  Malabsorption (inflammatory bowel diseases, celiac sprue, pancreatic disease, gastric resection or bypass)

Medications
  Glucocorticoids
  Aromatase inhibitors
  Gonadotropin-releasing hormone agonists
  Lithium
  Medroxyprogesterone acetate
  Chemotherapy and immunosuppressant
  Antiepileptics (phenobarbital, phenytoin, carbamazepine, valproate)
  Anticoagulants (heparin and coumadin)
  Thiazolidinediones
  Proton pump inhibitors
  Thyroid hormone (in supraphysiologic doses)
  Antiretrovirals (tenofovir, adefovir)
  Sodium-glucose co-transporter-2 inhibitors

Connective tissue disorders
  Osteogenesis imperfecta
  Marfan syndrome
  Ehlers-Danlos syndrome
  Homocystinuria

Hematologic disorders
  Multiple myeloma
  Leukemia and lymphoma
  Hemophilia
  Sickle cell disease
  Thalassemia
  Systemic mastocytosis

Miscellaneous
  Idiopathic hypercalciuria
  Immobilization
  Low physical activity
  Rheumatoid arthritis
  Chronic obstructive pulmonary disease
  Chronic kidney disease
  Congestive heart failure
  Human immunodeficiency virus and acquired immunodeficiency syndrome

Table 2	
FRAX tool	
Country of Origin	
Ethnicity	(US models only—white, black, Hispanic, and Asian)
Age	The model accepts ages between 40 and 90 y. If ages younger than or older than are entered, FRAX tool will compute probabilities at 40 and 90 y, respectively.
Sex	
Weight	(in kg)
Height	(in cm)
Previous fracture	(defined as fracture in adult life occurring spontaneously or fragility/low-trauma fracture)
Parental history of hip fracture	
Current smoking	
Glucocorticoid use	(defined as oral glucocorticoid use for more than 3 mo at a dosage of prednisolone $\geq$ 5 mg/d, or equivalent dose of other glucocorticoids)
Rheumatoid arthritis	
Secondary osteoporosis	(including type 1 diabetes mellitus, osteogenesis imperfecta, untreated longstanding hyperthyroidism, hypogonadism or premature menopause, chronic malnutrition or malabsorption, and chronic liver disease)
Alcohol use	($\geq$3 units of alcohol per day, the definition of a unit of alcohol depends on the country ranging from 8–10 g of alcohol)
Femoral neck bone mineral density (BMD) (or *T*-score)	In patients without a BMD test, the field should be left blank

The AACE 2020 guidelines recommend the following measures to prevent bone loss: adequate calcium intake of 1200 mg/d for women age $\geq$50 years (total intake including diet plus supplement, if needed), vitamin D3 supplementation if needed, with a daily dosage of 1000 to 2000 international units to maintain 25 OHD levels between 30 and 50 ng/mL, less than 2 servings of alcohol per day, limiting caffeine intake, smoking cessation, and maintaining an active lifestyle with recommended 30 minutes of weight-bearing exercise a day. Use of bone turnover markers in the initial evaluation and follow-up of osteoporosis patients can also be considered as elevated levels can predict more rapid rates of bone loss and higher fracture risk.[5]

Decision-Making on Pharmacologic Therapy

The goal of using pharmacologic therapies to treat low BMD or osteoporosis in postmenopausal women is to decrease the burden of major osteoporotic fractures. Pharmacologic therapy is indicated in patients with *T*-scores in the osteoporotic range and those with history of fragility fracture. However it is important to note that most fractures occur in patients with osteopenia or low bone mass (*T*-score between -1.0 and -2.5), as these individuals outnumber those with osteoporosis. Therefore, major osteoporosis guidelines[5,7] also recommend the treatment of patients with history of hip or vertebral fracture; or patients with osteopenia and a history of fragility fractures or with greater than or equal to 20% probability of major osteoporotic fracture or greater than or equal to 3% probability of a hip fracture in the next 10 years (or based on country-specific threshold) based on FRAX tool. In an update to the European Guidelines, patients are stratified into patients into low risk, high risk, and very high risk based on clinical factors such as age, sex, body mass index, prior fractures, with or without BMD.[8]

When starting treatment, it is appropriate to stratify patients by level of fracture risk (**Table 3**) because this may influence selection of initial treatment as well as the duration of therapy. Most patients are started on treatment because of high fracture risk. Some who are at very high fracture risk may require more aggressive treatment to achieve an acceptable level of fracture risk (**Tables 4** and **5**).

Several agents are approved by the Food and Drug Administration (FDA) for prevention and/or treatment of postmenopausal osteoporosis (**Table 6**). Head-to-head trial data are limited. Approved agents with efficacy to reduce hip, nonvertebral, and spine fractures including alendronate, denosumab, risedronate, and zoledronate are appropriate as initial therapy for most osteoporotic patients with high fracture risk. Abaloparatide, denosumab, romosozumab, teriparatide, and zoledronate should be considered for patients unable to use oral therapy and as initial therapy for patients at very high fracture risk (see **Tables 4** and **5**). These drugs also should be considered for those who have gastrointestinal problems and might not tolerate or absorb oral medication, and for patients who have trouble remembering to take oral medications or coordinating an oral bisphosphonate with other oral medications or daily routine. Ibandronate or raloxifene may be appropriate initial therapy in some cases for patients requiring drugs with spine-specific efficacy.

ANTIRESORPTIVE AGENTS
Bisphosphonates

Bisphosphonates are the most widely used class of medication for treatment of osteoporosis. These pyrophosphate analogues bind to hydroxyapatite crystals in the bone, inhibit function and recruitment of osteoclasts, and increase osteoclast apoptosis. Oral bioavailability is only 1% to 3%, but they have prolonged skeletal retention. In the United States, 4 bisphosphonates are available (alendronate, ibandronate, risedronate, and zoledronate), all available as generic preparations. Three of the 4 (alendronate, risedronate, and zoledronate) have evidence for broad-spectrum antifracture efficacy. A systematic review of trials published between 2005 and 2019 confirmed the vertebral fracture prevention efficacy of alendronate, risedronate, zoledronic acid, and ibandronate, compared with placebo.[10] Alendronate, risedronate, and zoledronic acid also reduce the risk of hip and other nonvertebral fractures.[11]

Oral bisphosphonates should be taken in the morning on an empty stomach (for maximal absorption) and with a full glass of water. Patients should be advised to remain upright for at least 30 minutes after ingestion. Bisphosphonates should be used with caution, if at all, in patients with reduced kidney function (glomerular filtration rate <30 mL/min for risedronate and ibandronate or <35 mL/min for alendronate). Before the administration of intravenous bisphosphonate, zoledronate, a creatinine clearance should be calculated based on the serum creatinine and actual body weight using the Cockcroft-Gault formula before each dose, and is not recommended for patients with creatinine clearance less than 35 mL/min.

Raloxifene

Raloxifene is a selective estrogen receptor modulator, with agonistic effects on bone. It is approved by the FDA for prevention and treatment of postmenopausal

Table 3
Risk stratification

Risk for Fractures	AACE/ACE 2020	Endocrine Society 2020	ESCEO/IOF 2019
Very high risk	Recent fracture (eg, within the past 12 mo) Fractures while on approved osteoporosis therapy History of multiple fractures Fractures while on drugs causing bone loss (eg, long-term glucocorticoids) Very low T-score (eg, <−3.0) High risk for falls History of very high fracture probability by FRAX	Multiple spine fractures BMD T-score at the hip or spine of −2.5 or below	Low, high, and very high risk based on FRAX/with or without BMD, refer to intervention thresholds[a] Examples: Prior fracture (of uncertain recency) Prior clinical vertebral fracture within the past 2 years Family history of hip fracture, exposure to glucocorticoids, exposure to higher than average doses of glucocorticoids B Bone mineral density (BMD) T-score at the femoral neck[b]
High risk	Patients who have been diagnosed with osteoporosis but are not at very high fracture risk as above	Prior spine or hip fracture BMD T-score at the hip or spine of −2.5 or below 10-y hip fracture risk ≥ 3%, or risk ofmajor osteoporoticfracture risk ≥ 20%	
Moderate risk		No prior hip or spine fractures BMD T-score at the hip and spine both above −2.5 10-y hip fracture risk < 3% or risk ofmajor osteoporotic fractures < 20%	
Low risk		No prior hip or spine fractures BMD T-score at the hip and spine both above −1.0 10-y hip fracture risk < 3%, and 10-yrisk ofmajor osteoporotic fractures < 20%	

Abbreviations: AACE/ACE, American Association of Clinical Endocrinologists/American College of Endocrinology; BMD, bone mineral density; ESCEO/IOF, European Society for Clinical and Economic Aspects of Osteoporosis and Osteoarthritis/International Osteoporosis Foundation.
[a] https://link.springer.com/article/10.1007/s00198-019-05176-3/figures/2.
[b] https://link.springer.com/article/10.1007/s00198-019-05176-3/tables/1.
Data from Refs.[5,7–9]

Table 4
Initial choice of agents

AACE/ACE 2020	Endocrine Society 2020	ESCEO/IOF 2019/2020
High risk: alendronate, risedronate, denosumab, zoledronate Very high risk: abaloparatide, denosumab, romosozumab, teriparatide, zoledronate	High risk: alendronate, risedronate, zoledronic acid, and ibandronate. Denosumab as alternative Very high risk: teriparatide, abaloparatide, romosozumab	High risk: oral bisphosphonates and other inhibitors of bone resorption Very high risk: anabolic agent followed by inhibitor of bone resorption

Abbreviations: AACE/ACE, American Association of Clinical Endocrinologists/American College of Endocrinology; ESCEO/IOF, European Society for Clinical and Economic Aspects of Osteoporosis and Osteoarthritis/International Osteoporosis Foundation.
Data from Refs.[5,7,8]

osteoporosis as well as for the reduction of risk of breast cancer in women with post-menopausal osteoporosis or at high risk of breast cancer. The major efficacy trial for raloxifene was the Multiple Outcomes of Raloxifene Evaluation (MORE) trial.[12] Ralox-ifene has been shown to reduce the risk of vertebral fracture. No significant difference in nonvertebral and hip fracture reduction was observed.

Calcitonin

Calcitonin is most useful as an alternative agent after an acute vertebral fracture given its systemic analgesic effects. It has modest effect on BMD and fracture reduction, and is recommended to be used with a stronger antiresorptive when possible.[13]

Estrogen

Although once considered the treatment of choice for postmenopausal osteoporosis, estrogen was never specifically approved for this use. Estrogen is approved by the FDA for prevention of postmenopausal osteoporosis with the added caveat, "when prescribing solely for the prevention of postmenopausal osteoporosis, therapy should only be considered for women at significant risk of osteoporosis and for whom non-estrogen medications are not considered to be appropriate." Current recommendations are to use estrogen for the relief of menopausal symptoms in the lowest dose necessary and for the shortest time possible.[5]

Table 5
Duration of therapy

AACE/ACE 2020	Endocrine Society 2020	ESCEO/IOF 2019/2020
Oral bisphosphonates for 5 y for high risk/up to 10 y for very high risk Zoledronate 3 y for high risk/up to 6 y for very high risk Assess fracture risk annually	Reassess fracture risk at 3–5 y	Reassess bisphosphonate use after 3–5 y Reassess after a new fracture

Abbreviations: AACE/ACE, American Association of Clinical Endocrinologists/American College of Endocrinology; ESCEO/IOF, European Society for Clinical and Economic Aspects of Osteoporosis and Osteoarthritis/International Osteoporosis Foundation.
Data from Refs.[5,7,9]

Table 6
Pharmacologic therapies: drugs approved by the U.S. Food and Drug Administration for treatment of postmenopausal osteoporosis

Antiresorptive Agents		Parathyroid Hormone Analogues		Romosozumab	
Bisphosphonates	10 mg PO daily	Teriparatide (Forteo)	20 μg SQ daily	Humanized monoclonal antibody against osteocyte-derived sclerostin (Evenity)	210 mg SQ monthly
Alendronate (Fosamax)	70 mg PO weekly	Abaloparatide (Tymlos)	80 μg SQ daily		
Risedronate(Actonel, Atelvia)	5 mg PO daily				
	35 mg PO weekly				
Ibandronate (Boniva)	150 mg PO monthly				
Zoledronate (Reclast)	2.5 mg PO daily				
Denosumab (Prolia)	150 mg PO monthly				
Selective estrogen agonists/antagonists	3 mg IV every 3 mo				
	5 mg IV once yearly				
Raloxifene (Evista)	60 mg SQ every 6 mo				
Estrogens	60 mg PO daily				
Multiple formulations	200 IU intranasally				
Calcitonin (Miacalcin, Fortical)	once daily or				
	100 IU SQ qod				

Abbreviations: IV, intravenous; PO, by mouth; qod, every other day; SQ, subcutaneous.

Denosumab

Denosumab is a human monoclonal antibody to Receptor activator of nuclear factor κB ligand (RANKL) that reversibly inhibits osteoclast-mediated bone resorption. RANKL binds to its receptor RANK on osteoclasts and osteoclast precursors acting as a key mediator of osteoclast differentiation, action, and survival. This process is regulated by a decoy receptor called osteoprotegrin that binds RANKL and prevents activation of osteoclasts. It is FDA approved for the treatment of osteoporosis in postmenopausal women, male osteoporosis, glucocorticoid-induced osteoporosis, and cancer treatment–induced bone loss.

Denosumab is administered as a 60-mg subcutaneous injection every 6 months. The effects of denosumab on bone remodeling, reflected in bone turnover markers, reverse after 6 months if the drug is not taken on schedule.[7] Case reports of multiple vertebral fractures on stopping denosumab therapy have been reported.[14] Drug holidays from denosumab are therefore not recommended because of this potential increased fracture risk. Although more data are needed to further elucidate the clinical impact of this phenomenon, patients should be informed about the importance of not missing a dose of denosumab and discontinuation of denosumab should be avoided without a proper treatment transition plan. The AACE/ACE Postmenopausal Osteoporosis Guidelines recommended that patients be transitioned with intravenous zoledronic acid or alternatively alendronate for 1 year. During this transition period, bone turnover markers and DXA can be followed and the patients closely monitored for evidence of rebound increase in bone resorption or multiple vertebral fractures[5] The ESCEO/IOF Guidelines also recommended the use of bisphosphonate after denosumab therapy to prevent an increase in vertebral fracture rate.[8]

ANABOLIC AGENTS
Teriparatide and Abaloparatide

Synthetic human parathyroid hormone (PTH) 1 to 34, or teriparatide (Forteo), is an anabolic agent that has been approved for the treatment of postmenopausal and male osteoporosis. The landmark trial in postmenopausal women was the Fracture Prevention Trial (FPT). In this randomized placebo-controlled trial (n = 1637) by Neer and colleagues,[15] postmenopausal women with at least 1 prior vertebral fracture, 20 µg teriparatide administered daily decreased the risk for new vertebral fractures by 65% and nonvertebral fragility fractures by 53%, with an increased BMD at lumbar spine by 9% and at femoral neck by 3% over a median follow-up period of 21 months.[15]

Abaloparatide (modified PTH-related peptide [PTHrP] 1–34) is approved by the FDA for the treatment of women with postmenopausal osteoporosis who are at high risk of fracture or have failed or been intolerant of previous osteoporosis therapy. It is also injected subcutaneously but it does not require refrigeration after use, compared with teriparatide.

The dose of abaloparatide is 80 µg daily, whereas teriparatide is given at 20 µg daily. It is recommended to measure serum calcium, PTH, and 25(OH)D levels, and alkaline phosphatase (to rule out Paget disease) before treatment with either medication.

Teriparatide was approved by the FDA in December of 2002 with a "black box" warning for potential increased risk of osteosarcoma, which was observed in a high percentage of rodents treated with high doses of teriparatide for most of their lifespan. A postmarketing surveillance program for evaluation of an association between osteosarcoma and treatment with teriparatide did not show any patients with osteosarcoma with prior teriparatide treatment.[16] Side effects of abaloparatide and teriparatide are similar and mild and transient and include nausea, orthostatic hypotension, and leg cramps. Elevated calcium level was also reported, but is usually mild, and transient. If serum calcium is measured, the blood should be drawn at least 16 hours after drug administration.

Teriparatide and abaloparatide are approved for treatment for up to 2 years for the reduction of vertebral and nonvertebral fractures. Once treatment course is completed, treatment with antiresorptive osteoporosis therapies to maintain bone density gain is recommended.

ROMOSOZUMAB

Romosozumab is a monoclonal antibody directed against sclerostin. Sclerostin is a product of the SOST gene that binds LRP5/6 and inhibits the Wnt signaling pathway and the differentiation of precursor cells into mature bone-forming osteoblasts. Blocking sclerostin binding to osteoblasts allows osteoblast activity to increase. Thus, inactivation or inhibition of sclerostin can lead to increased bone mass. The drug appears to have both an antiresorptive and anabolic effect.

Approval of romosozumab for postmenopausal women at high risk of fracture was based on 2 large trials. In the larger of the 2 trials (n = 7180),[17] patients were randomly assigned to receive subcutaneous injections of romosozumab (at a dosage of 210 mg) or placebo monthly for 12 months; thereafter, patients in each group received denosumab for 12 months, at a dosage of 60 mg, administered subcutaneously every 6 months. At 12 months, new vertebral fractures had occurred in 16 (0.5%) of 3321 patients in the romosozumab group, as compared with 59 (1.8%) of 3322 in the placebo group (representing a 73% lower risk with romosozumab; $P < .001$). Clinical fractures had occurred in 58 (1.6%) of 3589 patients in the romosozumab group, as compared with 90 (2.5%) of 3591 in the placebo group (a 36% lower risk with romosozumab; $P = .008$). Nonvertebral fractures had occurred in 56 (1.6%) of 3589 patients in the romosozumab group and in 75 (2.1%) of 3591 in the placebo group ($P = .10$). At 24 months, the rates of vertebral fractures were significantly lower in the romosozumab group than in the placebo group after each group made the transition to denosumab (0.6% [21 of 3325 patients] in the romosozumab group vs 2.5% [84 of 3327] in the placebo group, a 75% lower risk with romosozumab; $P < .001$).

In the other trial,[18] 4093 postmenopausal women with osteoporosis and a fragility fracture were assigned to receive monthly subcutaneous romosozumab (210 mg) or weekly oral alendronate (70 mg) in a blinded fashion for 12 months, followed by open-label alendronate in both groups. Over a period of 24 months, a 48% lower risk of new vertebral fractures was observed in the romosozumab-to-alendronate group (6.2% [127 of 2046 patients]) than in the alendronate-to-alendronate group (11.9% [243 of 2047 patients]) ($P < .001$). Clinical fractures occurred in 198 (9.7%) of 2046 patients in the romosozumab-to-alendronate group versus 266 (13.0%) of 2047 patients in the alendronate-to-alendronate group, representing a 27% lower risk with romosozumab ($P < .001$).

The recommended dosage is 210 mg monthly by subcutaneous injection for 12 months (**Table 7**). Women at high risk or with prior history of cardiovascular disease and stroke should not be considered for romosozumab pending further studies on cardiovascular risk associated with this treatment.

Romosozumab has also been studied in men but is not currently approved for male osteoporosis.

Table 7
Romosozumab use

AACE/ACE 2020	Endocrine Society 2020	ESCEO/IOF 2019
For very high risk patients, with prior fractures Follow with antiresorptive agent	Very high risk of fracture, such as those with severe osteoporosis (ie, low T-score < −2.5 and fractures) or multiple vertebral fractures Follow with antiresorptive agent	Not available at the time of publication

Abbreviations: AACE/ACE, American Association of Clinical Endocrinologists/American College of Endocrinology; ESCEO/IOF, European Society for Clinical and Economic Aspects of Osteoporosis and Osteoarthritis/International Osteoporosis Foundation.
   Data from Refs.[5,7,9]

SUMMARY

Significant advances have been made in the treatment of postmenopausal osteoporosis in the past decade. The latest guidelines from AACE, Endocrine Society, and the ESCEO/IOF have been updated and are mostly concordant in their recommendations as to risk stratification, initial therapy, and duration of treatment, as well as long-term follow-up patients.

CLINICS CARE POINTS

- When starting treatment, it is appropriate to stratify patients by level of fracture risk (low, high, and very high risk) to guide decision making in pharmacologic therapy such as selection of initial treatment and duration of therapy.
- Drug holidays from denosumab are not recommended due to potential increased fracture risk.
- Discontinuation of denosumab should be avoided without a proper treatment transition plan.
- Romosozumab, a monoclonal antibody directed against sclerostin, is now approved for use in treatment of postmenopausal osteoporosis.

DISCLOSURE

The author has nothing to disclose. Principal Investigator – Romosozumab ARCH Trial.

REFERENCES

1. Arceo-Mendoza RM, Camacho P. Prediction of fracture risk in patients with osteoporosis: a brief review. Womens Health (Lond). 2015;11(4):477–84.
2. Wright NC, Looker AC, Saag KG, et al. The recent prevalence of osteoporosis and low bone mass in the United States based on bone mineral density at the femoral neck or lumbar spine. J Bone Miner Res 2014;29(11):2520–6.
3. Burge R, Dawson-Hughes B, Solomon DH, et al. Incidence and economic burden of osteoporosis-related fractures in the United States, 2005-2025. J Bone Miner Res 2007;22(3):465–75.
4. Kanis JA. Diagnosis of osteoporosis and assessment of fracture risk. Lancet 2002;359(9321):1929–36.

5. Camacho PM, Petak SM, Binkley N, et al. American Association of Clinical Endocrinologists/American College of Endocrinology clinical practice guidelines for the diagnosis and treatment of postmenopausal osteoporosis-2020 update. Endocr Pract 2020;26(Suppl 1):1–46.

6. Kanis JA, Johansson H, Harvey NC, et al. A brief history of FRAX. Arch Osteoporos 2018;13(1):118.

7. Shoback D, Rosen CJ, Black DM, et al. Pharmacological management of osteoporosis in postmenopausal women: an endocrine society guideline update. J Clin Endocrinol Metab 2020;105(3):dgaa048.

8. Kanis JA, Harvey NC, McCloskey E, et al. Algorithm for the management of patients at low, high and very high risk of osteoporotic fractures. Osteoporos Int 2020;31(1):1–12. Erratum in: Osteoporos Int. 2020 Apr;31(4):797-798.

9. Kanis JA, Cooper C, Rizzoli R, et al. Scientific Advisory Board of the European Society for Clinical and Economic Aspects of Osteoporosis (ESCEO) and the Committees of Scientific Advisors and National Societies of the International Osteoporosis Foundation (IOF). Correction to: European guidance for the diagnosis and management of osteoporosis in postmenopausal women. Osteoporos Int 2019;30:3–44.

10. Crandall CJ, Newberry SJ, Diamant A, et al. Comparative effectiveness of pharmacologic treatments to prevent fractures: an updated systematic review. Ann Intern Med 2014;161(10):711–23.

11. Freemantle N, Cooper C, Diez-Perez A, et al. Results of indirect and mixed treatment comparison of fracture efficacy for osteoporosis treatments: a meta-analysis. Osteoporos Int 2013;24(1):209–17.

12. Ettinger B, Black DM, Mitlak BH, et al. Reduction of vertebral fracture risk in postmenopausal women with osteoporosis treated with raloxifene: results from a 3-year randomized clinical trial. Multiple Outcomes of Raloxifene Evaluation (MORE) Investigators [published correction appears in JAMA 1999 Dec 8;282(22):2124]. JAMA 1999;282(7):637–45.

13. Chestnut CH 3rd, Silverman S, Andriano K, et al. A randomized trial of nasal spray salmon calcitonin in postmenopausal women with established osteoporosis: the prevent recurrence of osteoporotic fractures study. PROOF Study Group. Am J Med 2000;109(4):267–76.

14. Anastasilakis AD, Evangelatos G, Makras P, et al. Rebound-associated vertebral fractures may occur in sequential time points following denosumab discontinuation: need for prompt treatment re-initiation. Bone Rep 2020;12:100267.

15. Neer RM, Arnaud CD, Zanchetta JR, et al. Effect of parathyroid hormone (1-34) on fractures and bone mineral density in postmenopausal women with osteoporosis. N Engl J Med 2001;344(19):1434–41.

16. Gilsenan A, Harding A, Kellier-Steele N, et al. The Forteo Patient Registry linkage to multiple state cancer registries: study design and results from the first 8 years. Osteoporos Int 2018;29(10):2335–43.

17. Cosman F, Crittenden DB, Adachi JD, et al. Romosozumab treatment in postmenopausal women with osteoporosis. N Engl J Med 2016;375(16):1532–43.

18. Saag KG, Petersen J, Brandi ML, et al. Romosozumab or alendronate for fracture prevention in women with osteoporosis. N Engl J Med 2017;377(15):1417–27.

Update on Approved Osteoporosis Therapies Including Combination and Sequential Use of Agents

Dominik Saul, MD[a,b,c], Matthew T. Drake, MD, PhD[a,b],*

KEYWORDS

- Osteoporosis • Postmenopausal • Bone • Anti-resorptive • Anabolic • Combination
- Sequential

KEY POINTS

- In postmenopausal women without contraindications, bisphosphonates remain the cornerstone of therapy for most patients.
- Although denosumab discontinuation is associated with rapid bone loss and increased risk for vertebral fractures, the optimal approach to denosumab discontinuation remains unknown.
- In patients at high risk for fracture, skeletal anabolic therapy is often the best option to limit the risk for future fractures.
- Romosozumab is a recently approved skeletal anabolic agent with a mechanism of action that differs from the other skeletal anabolic agents teriparatide and abaloparatide.
- Treatment with combination osteoporosis therapies is promising but may be a challenge for patient affordability.

INTRODUCTION

Osteoporosis is a multifactorial skeletal disorder. It is characterized by reduced bone mass and associated bone microarchitectural deterioration, which collectively lead to reduced bone strength and a heightened risk for fracture in affected patients.[1] Although most commonly recognized in women, there is overwhelming epidemiologic evidence that bone loss occurs in both women and men, with aging the most common

Grant support: D. Saul was supported by the Deutsche Forschungsgemeinschaft (DFG, German Research Foundation) – 413501650.

[a] Division of Endocrinology, Diabetes, Metabolism and Nutrition, Mayo Clinic, Rochester, MN, USA; [b] Robert and Arlene Kogod Center on Aging, Mayo Clinic, Rochester, MN, USA; [c] Department of Trauma Surgery, Orthopaedics and Plastic Surgery, University of Göttingen, Robert-Koch-Str. 40, Göttingen 37075, Germany

* Corresponding author. Division of Endocrinology and Kogod Center on Aging, Mayo Clinic College of Medicine, 200 First Street SW, Rochester, MN 55905.

E-mail address: Drake.Matthew@mayo.edu

risk factor.[2] It has been estimated that in the United States, roughly 50% of women and approximately 13% of men will suffer an osteoporosis-related fracture in their lifetime,[3] ultimately resulting in enormous societal and economic expenses.[4] Given space constraints and the inclusion within this larger issue of articles devoted to the topics of male osteoporosis and common secondary causes of osteoporosis, this article will focus primarily on postmenopausal osteoporosis. Unless otherwise noted (such as the section on estrogen/ selective estrogen receptor modulators SERMS), however, the information provided related to currently available bone anti-resorptive and anabolic agents is likely also applicable to men with osteoporosis based on expected common mechanisms of action in elderly women and men, although not all (eg, romosozumab) have been studied or approved for use in men.

Osteoporosis is most commonly identified by dual-energy x-ray absorptiometry (DXA) imaging, but can also be determined clinically in patients who have sustained a fragility fracture, defined as a fracture occurring from a mechanical force not normally anticipated to result in a fracture, such as a fall from a stranding height or less. Fortunately, multiple pharmacologic agents have been approved for the treatment of osteoporosis, with available evidence supporting both the clinical and cost-effectiveness of treatment initiation in patients who have previously suffered a fragility fracture, those with osteoporosis identified by DXA imaging, and those with osteopenia (low bone mass not meeting the DXA-based definition of osteoporosis) and additional associated clinical risk factors.[5] In this article, the authors will review currently available therapies, including more recent data on the use of combination and sequential therapies for the treatment of osteoporosis.

BONE ANTI-RESORPTIVE AGENTS
Bisphosphonates – General Properties

Bisphosphonates are chemically stable analogues of inorganic pyrophosphate that exhibit extremity high affinity for binding to hydroxyapatite, the inorganic component of bone. Early bisphosphonates (eg, clodronate, tiludronate, and etidronate) are non-nitrogen containing and cause osteoclast apoptosis by inhibiting ATP-dependent cellular processes within osteoclasts. Because of lower efficacy and a more limited therapeutic index, non-nitrogen-containing bisphosphates are now only infrequently used.[6]

In comparison, all subsequently developed bisphosphonates (alendronate, risedronate, ibandronate, and zoledronate) differ from their predecessors in that each has a nitrogen-containing sidechain. This fundamental structural difference results in even tighter binding to hydroxyapatite. Nitrogen-containing bisphosphonates also differ in the mechanism by which they induce osteoclast apoptosis, which occurs via inhibition of the farnesyl pyrophosphate synthase (FPPS) enzyme within osteoclasts.[7]

Finally, nitrogen-containing bisphosphonates are approved for delivery for the treatment of osteoporosis either orally (alendronate, risedronate, and ibandronate) or intravenously (ibandronate and zoledronate), with oral nitrogen-containing bisphosphonates 1% bioavailable compared to the 100% bioavailability of intravenously delivered nitrogen-containing bisphosphonates. Biologic half-lives for at least some of the nitrogen-containing bisphosphonates are estimated to be at least 5 years from time of administration.[8]

Alendronate
Alendronate was the first nitrogen-containing bisphosphonate approved in the United States based on data from the Fracture Intervention Trial (FIT) in which more than 2000 postmenopausal women aged at least 55 years with DXA-determined low bone

mineral density (BMD) at the femoral neck were randomized to receive either oral alendronate or placebo.[9] Alendronate reduced vertebral (by 47%) and hip (by 51%) fractures relative to placebo. Based on these data and data from the subsequent FIT-Long-term Extension study, in which subjects from this same cohort who had been treated with alendronate for 5 years in the parent FIT study were subsequently randomized to either continue alendronate therapy or changed to placebo for an additional 5years,[10] alendronate was found to be highly effective.

Risedronate

Risedronate was the second nitrogen-containing bisphosphonate to receive US Food and Drug Administration (FDA) approval, which occurred after documentation of clinical efficacy in the Vertebral Efficacy with Risedronate Therapy (VERT) trial, in which nearly 2500 postmenopausal women aged under 85 years were randomized to risedronate or placebo.[11] In VERT, 3 years of risedronate treatment reduced vertebral (by 41%) and nonvertebral (by 39%) fractures, findings that were confirmed in a parallel study conducted outside the United States.[12]

Ibandronate

Ibandronate was the third nitrogen-containing oral bisphosphonate approved in the United States, based on data from the BONE study, a trial in which nearly 3000 postmenopausal women were randomized to either ibandronate or placebo treatment for 3 years.[13] Comparable efficacy to alendronate and risedronate for reduction of vertebral fractures was noted, although unlike alendronate and risedronate, ibandronate did not show efficacy for prevention of nonvertebral or hip fractures. Finally, unlike both alendronate and risedronate, ibandronate is FDA approved in both oral and intravenous formations for the treatment and prevention of osteoporosis.

Zoledronate

As an intravenous nitrogen-containing bisphosphonate, zoledronate is approved in the United States as a once-yearly intravenous infusion for the treatment of osteoporosis. When provided annually for 3 years in the Health Outcomes and Reduced Incidence with Zoledronic Acid Once Yearly (HORIZON) trial in nearly 4000 postmenopausal women, zoledronate reduced the incidence of vertebral (70%), nonvertebral (25%), and hip (41%) fractures relative to placebo.[14]

More recent studies have documented that zoledronate dosing provided at greater than 1-year intervals remains effective for many patients. Thus, treatment of 2000 postmenopausal women aged 65 years and older with osteopenia at the hip by DXA imaging with zoledronate or placebo infusions at 18 month intervals over 6 years resulted in a 37% reduction in fragility fractures, including a 55% decrease in vertebral fractures, in subjects treated with zoledronate.[15] Further analysis of this cohort showed that beyond the documented skeletal effects described, zoledronate treatment was also associated with reduced rates of vascular events, cancer incidence (both breast and nonbreast cancers), and a trend toward reduced mortality,[16] suggesting that future studies designed to examine a role for zoledronate therapy in nonskeletal outcomes may be warranted. Finally, a study of postmenopausal women with DXA-documented osteopenia provided with a single dose of zoledronate at baseline and then again 5.5 years later showed no loss of bone mass after 5.5 additional years (11 years in total), suggesting that very infrequent zoledronate dosing is highly efficacious for maintenance of bone mass, although fracture outcomes could not be statistically evaluated because of the small number of subjects enrolled.[17]

As will be discussed, the optimal role for bisphosphonate (particularly zoledronate) therapy in relation to other pharmacologic agents continues to be an area of active investigation.

Denosumab

Denosumab is a humanized monoclonal antibody that binds to and inhibits the osteoclast-activating factor receptor activator of nuclear factor kappa-B ligand (RANKL). Denosumab was approved by the FDA based on the results of the Fracture Reduction Evaluation of Denosumab in Osteoporosis Every Six Months (FREEDOM) trial, in which nearly 8000 women with postmenopausal osteoporosis were treated for 3 years with subcutaneous denosumab or placebo provided every 6 months.[18] Relative to placebo, denosumab reduced the incidence of vertebral (by 68%), nonvertebral (by 20%), and hip (by 40%) fractures.

Although not recognized at the time of FDA approval, discontinuation of denosumab therapy (or prolongation of the normal 6-month interval at which denosumab is provided) is associated with a rapid increase in biochemical markers of bone resorption, a rapid decline in bone mass such that BMD returns to pretreatment levels within 12 months of denosumab discontinuation, and a marked increase in the risk for vertebral fracture (including multiple vertebral fractures) occurrence, particularly in subjects with prior vertebral fractures.[19] Having received treatment with bisphosphonate before denosumab initiation is associated with a reduction in the rebound osteoclast-mediated bone resorption that occurs with denosumab discontinuation, but whether this attenuation limits either BMD loss or fracture development following denosumab cessation is unclear.[20] Apart from denosumab continuation at an every 6-month dosing interval once initiated, an approach based on the FREEDOM open-label extension[21] and bone biopsy analyses[22] appears to be safe for up to 10 years following denosumab initiation when used for the treatment of osteoporosis. It is recommended that patients who wish or need to discontinue denosumab therapy should be transitioned to an alternative anti-resorptive therapy beginning 6 months after their last denosumab injection in order to limit the negative skeletal effects associated with denosumab discontinuation.[20] The optimal anti-resorptive (either oral or intravenous bisphosphonate) and dosing regimen to prevent denosumab discontinuation-associated rebound osteoclastogenesis and bone loss remains unknown, and is an active area of investigation. To date, early data suggest that infusion of a single dose of zoledronate 6 months or 9 months after the last denosumab injection is insufficient to prevent this increase in bone resorption,[23] whereas transition to alendronate may be partially able to mitigate the bone loss associated with denosumab discontinuation.[24]

ESTROGEN/SELECTIVE ESTROGEN RECEPTOR MODULATORS

Ovarian failure results in a rapid decline in circulating estrogen (primarily estradiol) levels and heralds the menopausal onset, and with it rapid bone loss. Pharmacologic treatment with oral or topical estrogen functions both as an anti-resorptive and anabolic within the skeleton.[25] However, because of nonskeletal concerns raised in the Women's Health Initiative trial, the use of estrogens (both oral and topical) for the prevention and treatment of osteoporosis has declined precipitously.

The SERM raloxifene is approved by the FDA for the prevention and treatment of postmenopausal osteoporosis, although its use in clinical practice is commonly reserved for patients with contraindications to other more potent agents, or for postmenopausal women who prefer a simultaneous approach to limit breast cancer risk.[26]

More recently, a combination of the SERM bazedoxifene with conjugated estrogens was approved for the prevention of postmenopausal osteoporosis.[26]

BONE ANABOLIC AGENTS

Anti-resorptive agents function to limit the activity of bone-resorbing osteoclasts. Accordingly, however, they represent only 1 side of a 2-edged sword that can be wielded in the battle against osteoporosis. On the other side are skeletal anabolic agents that function by stimulating osteoblast recruitment and activity in order to increase bone mass. To date, 3 agents have been approved for the treatment of osteoporosis, and will be discussed.

Both teriparatide (representing the amino-terminal 34 amino acids of the endogenous parathyroid hormone [PTH] molecule) and abaloparatide (a 34-amino acid analogue with 76% homology to PTH-related protein) exert their activities by binding to the G-protein coupled PTH 1 receptor (PTH1R). Although perpetual activation of the PTH1R (as occurs in primary hyperparathyroidism) leads to bone resorption, intermittent PTH1R stimulation results in bone formation. As a result of the coupling that occurs between osteoblasts and osteoclasts,[27] both osteoblast-mediated bone formation and osteoclast-mediated bone resorption are increased with intermittent administration of teriparatide and abaloparatide, although the relative increase in osteoclast-mediated bone resorption appears to be less in response to abaloparatide treatment.[28] Importantly, this coupling that occurs between osteoblasts and osteoclasts is likely, at least in part, the reason that all currently available skeletal anabolic agents (teriparatide, abaloparatide, and romosozumab) require subsequent administration of a skeletal anti-resorptive agent to maximize the skeletal increases accrued with anabolic therapy, because of the anticipated rebound increase of bone resorption after anabolic agent withdrawal.[29]

TERIPARATIDE

As first described 2 decades ago in a study of approximately 1600 postmenopausal women, once-daily teriparatide administration for a median of 21 months reduced vertebral (by 65%) and nonvertebral (by 53%) fractures and increased lumbar spine (by 9%) and femoral neck (by 3%) BMD compared with placebo. These results led to the 2002 FDA approval of teriparatide for the treatment of postmenopausal osteoporosis, and subsequent European Medicines Agency (EMA) approval in 2003.[30]

In recent years, there have been several new insights into the clinical utility of teriparatide. In the VERO trial, more than 1300 postmenopausal women with at least 2 moderate or 1 severe vertebral fracture(s) and a BMD T-score no more than −1.5 were randomized to 24 months of treatment with daily teriparatide plus weekly oral placebo or daily placebo plus weekly oral risedronate. In the group that received teriparatide, new radiographic vertebral (by 56%), clinical (by 52%), and non-vertebral (by 34%) fractures were reduced.[31] Although a potential criticism related to the study design is the parenteral versus oral treatment administration of the study agents, the treatment compliance of 72% was identical in both groups and was therefore felt to be sufficient to draw conclusions from the generated data.[32] Therefore, in a group of postmenopausal women at high fracture risk, teriparatide treatment appeared superior when compared with oral bisphosphonate therapy for the clinically important outcome of fracture.

Although medication-related osteonecrosis of the jaw (MRONJ) has become less common in clinical practice with more judicious use of anti-resorptive (primarily bisphosphonates and denosumab) agents, it remains a challenge to treat when it does occur.[33] In a placebo-controlled, double-blind randomized trial of 34 subjects, treatment with daily teriparatide for 8 weeks led to greater resolution of MRONJ lesions (odds ratio 0.15 for teriparatide vs 0.40 for placebo), suggesting that teriparatide may be of benefit for the treatment of this otherwise difficult to manage condition.[34]

ABALOPARATIDE

Abaloparatide received FDA approval in 2017, but was denied approval in Europe by the EMA because of the concerns that the phase 3 Abaloparatide Comparator Trial in Vertebral Endpoints (ACTIVE) study (used for FDA approval in the United States) did not satisfactorily demonstrate that abaloparatide prevented nonvertebral fractures in postmenopausal women, as well as concerns related to the medication's effect on heart rate and palpitations.[35]

In the ACTIVE study, nearly 2500 women were randomized to treatment for 18 months with placebo, abaloparatide, or teriparatide. Relative to placebo, abaloparatide reduced vertebral (by 86%) and nonvertebral (by 43%) fractures and increased mean differences in BMD at the lumbar spine (+10.37%), femoral neck (+4.01%), and total hip (+4.25%) compared with placebo.[36] However, the overall vertebral fracture rates (4/690 subjects in the abaloparatide group vs 30/711 subjects in the placebo group), particularly in the placebo group, were much lower than expected, raising potential concerns about the study design.[37] In the ACTIVExtend study, the abaloparatide- and placebo-treated subjects were treated for an additional 24 months with alendronate, with a continued 87% vertebral fracture relative risk reduction in the group previously treated with abaloparatide.[38]

Numerous subsequent post hoc and subgroup analyses of the ACTIVE and ACTIVExtend studies also have been performed recently. Results from these studies demonstrate that

- In postmenopausal women, initial abaloparatide treatment may be associated with a greater reduction in vertebral fractures than alendronate treatment[39]
- The effects of abaloparatide in younger postmenopausal women (aged 49–64 years) were similar to those seen in the larger cohort of older women studied in the trials[40]
- Postmenopausal women with type 2 diabetes responded similarly to abaloparatide compared to women without type 2 diabetes[41]
- No safety signals were identified in patients with mild-to-moderate renal dysfunction who received abaloparatide, suggesting that no adjustment to abaloparatide dosing is required for patients with mild-to-moderate renal impairment[42]

ROMOSOZUMAB

Unlike the skeletal anabolic agents teriparatide and abaloparatide, which are peptides delivered by daily subcutaneous injection, romosozumab is a humanized monoclonal antibody that binds and thereby inhibits sclerostin, an osteocyte-secreted Wnt signaling pathway inhibitor. Although a potent bone anabolic agent, continued delivery of romosozumab is also associated with simultaneous inhibition of bone resorption likely via inhibition of RANKL release from osteocytes.[28]

Based on data from the international, double-blind FRAME trial, in which nearly 7200 postmenopausal women were randomized to monthly treatment with romosozumab or placebo for 12 months, romosozumab received approval in 2019 from both the FDA and EMA for the treatment of postmenopausal women with osteoporosis. Romosozumab treatment reduced vertebral (by 73%) and clinical (by 36%) fractures relative to placebo over 12 months of treatment, results that were maintained during months 13 to 24 when subjects in both the romosozumab and placebo cohorts were transitioned to denosumab.[43,44] Notably, because of concerns related to a potentially slight increase in risk for adverse cardiovascular events in subjects treated with romosozumab, a history of myocardial infarction or cerebrovascular accident within the preceding year is considered a contraindication to treatment initiation.[45]

In the ARCH study, which randomized nearly 4100 postmenopausal women with osteoporosis and a fragility fracture to romosozumab or weekly alendronate for 12 months, followed by alendronate for an additional 12 months, upfront romosozumab therapy decreased vertebral (by 48%), clinical (by 27%), nonvertebral (by 19%), and hip (by 38%) fractures compared with placebo.[45,46]

Similar to the results shown in postmenopausal women, treatment of men with osteoporosis aged 55 to 90 years in the BRIDGE study with romosozumab or placebo for 12 months led to significant improvement in BMD at both the lumbar spine (+10.9%) and total hip (+3.0%) in men who received romosozumab. Importantly, there was a numerical imbalance in adjudicated cardiovascular serious adverse events in the romosozumab (4.9%) versus placebo (2.5%) cohorts, respectively.[47]

COMBINATION AND SEQUENTIAL THERAPY
Combination Therapy

Combination therapy involves the use of a bone anabolic agent provided in conjunction with an anti-resorptive agent. To date, combination therapies have only been evaluated in studies that have used changes in BMD (ie, not fracture) as a study endpoint.

In a study of more than 400 postmenopausal women with osteoporosis, combining teriparatide with a single dose of concomitantly provided zoledronate did not increase lumbar spine BMD more than treatment with teriparatide alone over 12 months.[48] Likewise, the combination of teriparatide and denosumab has been previously evaluated in the Denosumab and Teriparatide Administration (DATA) trial, in which denosumab and teriparatide provided concomitantly was compared with either treatment alone in nearly 100 postmenopausal women with osteoporosis studied over 2 years.[49] Although combination treatment increased BMD more than treatment with either agent alone, markers of bone turnover in the combination group more closely resembled those in the denosumab alone group, suggesting that when provided together denosumab may at least partially blunt the skeletal anabolic effect of teriparatide.

More recently, teriparatide was evaluated in combination with denosumab in the DATA High Dose (DATA-HD) trial, an open-label phase 4 study in which postmenopausal women were randomized to treatment with either standard-dose (20 µg; N = 39 subjects) or high-dose (40 µg; N = 37 subjects) teriparatide for 9 months. Importantly, standard dose denosumab therapy was initiated 3 months after teriparatide initiation in both groups and was continued for 12 months. Mean differences in the increases seen at the lumbar spine (+8.1%), femoral neck (+2.5%), and total hip (+2.2%) were all statistically greater in subjects who received high dose-teriparatide, although neither treatment tolerability nor safety could be assessed because of the limited study size.[50]

Although combination therapy may be of benefit for some postmenopausal women, at present, the data would suggest that for most patients (and in particular those who are treatment naïve), initiation of skeletal anabolic therapy without concomitant anti-resorptive therapy is likely the best option.

Sequential Therapy

Both in the setting of treatment failure and while caring for patients with severe osteoporosis and high fracture risk, changes in therapy are frequently needed. Although treatment may involve changing from one anti-resorptive agent to a second anti-resorptive agent, any sequence of therapies is in theory possible. As seen with studies of combination therapies, however, most studies that have examined sequential therapies have used surrogate markers for fracture (namely changes in BMD and biochemical markers of bone turnover) as endpoints.

Anti-resorptive Agent Followed by Anti-resorptive Agent

In a double-blind study of nearly 650 postmenopausal women with DXA-determined osteoporosis previously treated with alendronate for an average of 6.3 years and randomized to treatment with denosumab or zoledronate for an additional 12 months, BMD increases at the lumbar spine, femoral neck, and total hip, and declines in biochemical markers of bone turnover were greater in denosumab-treated subjects.[51]

Anti-resorptive Agent Followed by Anti-resorptive or Anabolic Agents

A recent study retrospectively evaluated the comparative effectiveness of 2 years of treatment with teriparatide or denosumab, provided as FDA approved, in 215 patients previously maintained on long-term bisphosphonate therapy (median duration 7.0 years). When compared with patients who received denosumab, teriparatide-treated patients displayed higher annualized BMD increases at the spine (+1.3%), but lower BMD changes at the femur neck (−1.1%), and total hip (−2.2%).[52] Collectively, these findings highlight the potential for loss of bone mass at the hip when switching from bisphosphonate to teriparatide therapy, a consideration of particular importance in individuals deemed to be at high risk for hip fracture.

Anti-resorptive Therapy Followed by Anabolic Therapy

When considering anti-resorptive versus anabolic therapy, the sequence in which each is provided can have profound effects on anticipated increases in BMD.[53] Although in general it is preferable to provide anabolic therapy prior to anti-resorptive therapy, in clinical practice this is not always possible because of insurance company mandates that frequently require prior anti-resorptive agent treatment failure.

In the VERO trial, in which postmenopausal women with osteoporosis were randomized to treatment for 24 months with daily teriparatide plus weekly oral placebo or daily placebo plus weekly oral risedronate, roughly 60% of subjects in both the teriparatide treatment and risedronate treatment groups had received bisphosphonate treatment for a median of 3.7 years prior to study enrollment. In a preplanned subgroup analysis, teriparatide treatment was associated with a significantly lower risk for new vertebral (by 56%) and clinical (by 34%) fractures, with antifracture efficacy for teriparatide similar in patients who had previously received bisphosphonate treatment and in those who had not.[31]

In comparison, treatment with denosumab prior to teriparatide, as studied in the DATA-Switch study in which postmenopausal women with osteoporosis were treated with denosumab for 2 years prior to changing to teriparatide, resulted in a marked increase in biochemical markers of bone turnover and a decline in BMD at the femoral neck and total hip.[54]

Finally, the transition from bisphosphonate therapy to either romosozumab or teriparatide was recently examined in STRUCTURE, a study in which nearly 450 women with postmenopausal osteoporosis who had previously received bisphosphonate therapy for an average of greater than 6 years were randomized to 12 months of treatment with romosozumab or teriparatide.[55] Relative to changes in BMD previously documented to occur in treatment-naïve women, BMD increases were blunted in both cohorts, although increases at the lumbar spine, femoral neck, and total hip were significantly greater in women treated with romosozumab.

Anabolic Therapy Followed by Anti-resorptive Therapy

As noted previously, all currently available skeletal anabolic agents must be followed by anti-resorptive therapy to maximize the skeletal increases accrued with anabolic therapy and prevent bone resorption following anabolic agent discontinuation.

This effect has been demonstrated most frequently in studies of teriparatide, in which subsequent treatment with alendronate[56] or denosumab[54] resulted in sustained increases and subsequent maintenance in BMD at both the lumbar spine and hip sites.

Likewise, in the ACTIVExtend study, both the abaloparatide- and placebo-treated cohorts were provided with an additional 24 months of treatment with alendronate, with the 87% vertebral fracture relative risk reduction maintained in the abaloparatide-treated group.[38]

Finally, several studies have now examined the effect of anti-resorptive therapy following romosozumab discontinuation. In the FRAME study of nearly 7200 postmenopausal women, treatment with romosozumab or placebo for 12 months followed by denosumab increased BMD in both groups, a difference that was maintained at the 24-month time point. Likewise, in the ARCH study, nearly 4100 postmenopausal women with high fracture risk were randomized to treatment with romosozumab versus alendronate alone for 1 year, followed by alendronate for an additional year in both groups. Treatment with alendronate maintained the romosozumab-mediated increase in BMD and the reduction in vertebral fracture risk.[57]

SUMMARY

Although postmenopausal osteoporosis is associated with tremendous morbidity and societal cost, efforts to stem the growing tide of fractures in the aging population have lost traction, particularly over the past decade. However, much work over the past several decades has provided a plethora of pharmacologic agents with demonstrated efficacy for maintaining or improving bone mass and reducing fracture risk through the targeting of bone resorbing osteoclasts and/or bone forming osteoblasts. Although current armamentarium is predicated on a foundation of ever-increasing understanding of bone pathobiology that has been built over decades, it is likely that future treatments may be based on therapies specific for the key signaling pathways than have gone awry in individual patients. Until such approaches are available, however, the approach to each patient must reflect current understanding of each patient's individualized risk factors, using a patient-centered approach to optimize care decisions and limit the risks of bone loss and fracture by employing available agents to maximum effect based on currently available data.

CLINICS CARE POINTS

- Osteoporosis can be diagnosed by BMD testing or by a history of fragility fracture.

- Although studied most extensively in postmenopausal women, bone anti-resorptive (bisphosphonates and denosumab) and anabolic (eg, teriparatide, abaloparatide, and romosozumab) therapies are expected to work equally well in men, as their mechanisms of action are not sex specific.
- Skeletal anabolic therapy must be followed by anti-resorptive therapy to prevent loss of bone mass accrued with skeletal anabolic treatment.
- BMD increases are generally greater when anabolic therapy is followed by anti-resorptive therapy, versus when anti-resorptive therapy is followed by anabolic therapy.

DISCLOSURE

Neither D. Saul nor M.T. Drake have any relevant disclosures.

REFERENCES

1. NIH Consensus Development Panel on Osteoporosis Prevention, Diagnosis, and Therapy. Osteoporosis prevention, diagnosis, and therapy. JAMA 2001;285(6): 785–95.
2. Drake MT, Clarke BL, Lewiecki EM. The pathophysiology and treatment of osteoporosis. Clin Ther 2015;37(8):1837–50.
3. Rosen CJ. The epidemiology and pathogenesis of osteoporosis. In: Feingold KR, Anawalt B, Boyce A, et al, editors. Endotext. South Dartmouth (MA): MDText.com, Inc.; 2020.
4. Williams SA, Chastek B, Sundquist K, et al. Economic burden of osteoporotic fractures in US managed care enrollees. Am J Manag Care 2020;26(5):e142–9.
5. Tosteson ANA, Melton LJ, Dawson-Hughes B, et al. Cost-effective osteoporosis treatment thresholds: the United States perspective. Osteoporos Int 2008;19(4): 437–47.
6. Drake MT, Clarke BL, Khosla S. Bisphosphonates: mechanism of action and role in clinical practice. Mayo Clin Proc 2008;83(9):1032–45.
7. Baron R, Ferrari S, Russell RGG. Denosumab and bisphosphonates: different mechanisms of action and effects. Bone 2011;48(4):677–92.
8. Khan SA, Kanis JA, Vasikaran S, et al. Elimination and biochemical responses to intravenous alendronate in postmenopausal osteoporosis. J Bone Miner Res 1997;12(10):1700–7.
9. Black DM, Cummings SR, Karpf DB, et al. Randomised trial of effect of alendronate on risk of fracture in women with existing vertebral fractures. Fracture Intervention Trial Research Group. Lancet 1996;348(9041):1535–41.
10. Black DM, Schwartz AV, Ensrud KE, et al. Effects of continuing or stopping alendronate after 5 years of treatment: the Fracture Intervention Trial Long-term Extension (FLEX): a randomized trial. JAMA 2006;296(24):2927–38.
11. Harris ST, Watts NB, Genant HK, et al. Effects of risedronate treatment on vertebral and nonvertebral fractures in women with postmenopausal osteoporosis: a randomized controlled trial. Vertebral Efficacy With Risedronate Therapy (VERT) Study Group. JAMA 1999;282(14):1344–52.
12. Reginster J, Minne HW, Sorensen OH, et al. Randomized trial of the effects of risedronate on vertebral fractures in women with established postmenopausal osteoporosis. Vertebral Efficacy with Risedronate Therapy (VERT) Study Group. Osteoporos Int 2000;11(1):83–91.

13. Chesnut CH, Skag A, Christiansen C, et al. Effects of oral ibandronate administered daily or intermittently on fracture risk in postmenopausal osteoporosis. J Bone Miner Res 2004;19(8):1241–9.
14. Black DM, Delmas PD, Eastell R, et al. Once-yearly zoledronic acid for treatment of postmenopausal osteoporosis. N Engl J Med 2007;356(18):1809–22.
15. Reid IR, Horne AM, Mihov B, et al. Fracture prevention with zoledronate in older women with osteopenia. N Engl J Med 2018;379(25):2407–16.
16. Reid IR, Horne AM, Mihov B, et al. Effects of zoledronate on cancer, cardiac events, and mortality in osteopenic older women. J Bone Miner Res 2020; 35(1):20–7.
17. Grey A, Horne A, Gamble G, et al. Ten years of very infrequent zoledronate therapy in older women: an open-label extension of a randomized trial. J Clin Endocrinol Metab 2020;105(4):dgaa062.
18. Cummings SR, San Martin J, McClung MR, et al. Denosumab for prevention of fractures in postmenopausal women with osteoporosis. N Engl J Med 2009; 361(8):756–65.
19. Cummings SR, Ferrari S, Eastell R, et al. Vertebral fractures after discontinuation of denosumab: a post hoc analysis of the randomized placebo-controlled FREEDOM trial and its extension. J Bone Miner Res 2018;33(2):190–8.
20. Tsourdi E, Zillikens MC, Meier C, et al. Fracture risk and management of discontinuation of denosumab therapy: a systematic review and position statement by ECTS. J Clin Endocrinol Metab 2020. https://doi.org/10.1210/clinem/dgaa756.
21. Bone HG, Wagman RB, Brandi ML, et al. 10 years of denosumab treatment in postmenopausal women with osteoporosis: results from the phase 3 randomised FREEDOM trial and open-label extension. Lancet Diabetes Endocrinol 2017;5(7): 513–23.
22. Dempster DW, Brown JP, Fahrleitner-Pammer A, et al. Effects of long-term denosumab on bone histomorphometry and mineralization in women with postmenopausal osteoporosis. J Clin Endocrinol Metab 2018;103(7):2498–509.
23. Sølling AS, Harsløf T, Langdahl B. Treatment with zoledronate subsequent to denosumab in osteoporosis: a randomized trial. J Bone Miner Res 2020;35(10): 1858–70.
24. Kendler D, Chines A, Clark P, et al. Bone mineral density after transitioning from denosumab to alendronate. J Clin Endocrinol Metab 2020;105(3):e255–64.
25. Khastgir G, Studd J, Holland N, et al. Anabolic effect of estrogen replacement on bone in postmenopausal women with osteoporosis: histomorphometric evidence in a longitudinal study. J Clin Endocrinol Metab 2001;86(1):289–95.
26. Pinkerton JV. Hormone therapy for postmenopausal women. N Engl J Med 2020; 382(5):446–55.
27. Weivoda MM, Chew CK, Monroe DG, et al. Identification of osteoclast-osteoblast coupling factors in humans reveals links between bone and energy metabolism. Nat Commun 2020;11(1):87.
28. Langdahl B. Treatment of postmenopausal osteoporosis with bone-forming and antiresorptive treatments: Combined and sequential approaches. Bone 2020;115516.
29. Lukert BP. Which drug next? sequential therapy for osteoporosis. J Clin Endocrinol Metab 2020;105(3):dgaa007.
30. Neer RM, Arnaud CD, Zanchetta JR, et al. Effect of parathyroid hormone (1-34) on fractures and bone mineral density in postmenopausal women with osteoporosis. N Engl J Med 2001;344(19):1434–41.

31. Kendler DL, Marin F, Zerbini CAF, et al. Effects of teriparatide and risedronate on new fractures in post-menopausal women with severe osteoporosis (VERO): a multicentre, double-blind, double-dummy, randomised controlled trial. Lancet 2018;391(10117):230–40.

32. Liel Y. Teriparatide vs risedronate for osteoporosis. Lancet 2018;391(10133): 1895.

33. Khan AA, Morrison A, Hanley DA, et al. Diagnosis and management of osteonecrosis of the jaw: a systematic review and international consensus. J Bone Miner Res 2015;30(1):3–23.

34. Sim I-W, Borromeo GL, Tsao C, et al. Teriparatide promotes bone healing in medication-related osteonecrosis of the jaw: a placebo-controlled, randomized trial. J Clin Oncol 2020;JCO1902192. https://doi.org/10.1200/JCO.19.02192.

35. European Medicines Agency. Assessment report Eladynos: international non-proprietary name: abaloparatide. [Procedure No. EMEA/H/C/004157/0000] 2018. Available at: https://www.ema.europa.eu/en/documents/assessment-report/eladynos-epar-refusal-public-assessment-report_en.pdf. Accessed July 10, 2020.

36. Miller PD, Hattersley G, Riis BJ, et al. Effect of abaloparatide vs placebo on new vertebral fractures in postmenopausal women with osteoporosis: a randomized clinical trial. JAMA 2016;316(7):722–33.

37. Cappola AR, Shoback DM. Osteoporosis therapy in postmenopausal women with high risk of fracture. JAMA 2016;316(7):715–6.

38. Bone HG, Cosman F, Miller PD, et al. ACTIVExtend: 24 months of alendronate after 18 months of abaloparatide or placebo for postmenopausal osteoporosis. J Clin Endocrinol Metab 2018;103(8):2949–57.

39. Leder BZ, Mitlak B, Hu M, et al. Effect of abaloparatide vs alendronate on fracture risk reduction in postmenopausal women with osteoporosis. J Clin Endocrinol Metab 2020;105(3):938–43.

40. Saag KG, Williams SA, Wang Y, et al. Effect of abaloparatide on bone mineral density and fracture incidence in a subset of younger postmenopausal women with osteoporosis at high risk for fracture. Clin Ther 2020;42(6):1099–107.e1.

41. Dhaliwal R, Hans D, Hattersley G, et al. Abaloparatide in postmenopausal women with osteoporosis and type 2 diabetes: a post hoc analysis of the ACTIVE Study. JBMR Plus 2020;4(4):e10346.

42. Bilezikian JP, Hattersley G, Mitlak BH, et al. Abaloparatide in patients with mild or moderate renal impairment: results from the ACTIVE phase 3 trial. Curr Med Res Opin 2019;35(12):2097–102.

43. Cosman F, Crittenden DB, Adachi JD, et al. Romosozumab treatment in postmenopausal women with osteoporosis. N Engl J Med 2016;375(16):1532–43.

44. Kalyan S. Romosozumab treatment in postmenopausal osteoporosis. N Engl J Med 2017;376(4):395–7.

45. Saag KG, Petersen J, Brandi ML, et al. Romosozumab or alendronate for fracture prevention in women with osteoporosis. N Engl J Med 2017;377(15):1417–27.

46. Tsourdi E, Rachner TD, Hofbauer LC. Romosozumab versus alendronate and fracture risk in women with osteoporosis. N Engl J Med 2018;378(2):194–6.

47. Lewiecki EM, Blicharski T, Goemaere S, et al. A Phase III randomized placebo-controlled trial to evaluate efficacy and safety of romosozumab in men with osteoporosis. J Clin Endocrinol Metab 2018;103(9):3183–93.

48. Cosman F, Eriksen EF, Recknor C, et al. Effects of intravenous zoledronic acid plus subcutaneous teriparatide rhPTH(1-34) in postmenopausal osteoporosis. J Bone Miner Res 2011;26(3):503–11.

49. Leder BZ, Tsai JN, Uihlein AV, et al. Two years of denosumab and teriparatide administration in postmenopausal women with osteoporosis (The DATA Extension Study): a randomized controlled trial. J Clin Endocrinol Metab 2014;99(5): 1694–700.

50. Tsai JN, Lee H, David NL, et al. Combination denosumab and high dose teriparatide for postmenopausal osteoporosis (DATA-HD): a randomised, controlled phase 4 trial. Lancet Diabetes Endocrinol 2019;7(10):767–75.

51. Miller PD, Pannacciulli N, Brown JP, et al. Denosumab or zoledronic acid in postmenopausal women with osteoporosis previously treated with oral bisphosphonates. J Clin Endocrinol Metab 2016;101(8):3163–70.

52. Lyu H, Zhao SS, Yoshida K, et al. Comparison of teriparatide and denosumab in patients switching from long-term bisphosphonate use. J Clin Endocrinol Metab 2019;104(11):5611–20.

53. Cosman F, Nieves JW, Dempster DW. Treatment sequence matters: anabolic and antiresorptive therapy for osteoporosis. J Bone Miner Res 2017;32(2):198–202.

54. Leder BZ, Tsai JN, Uihlein AV, et al. Denosumab and teriparatide transitions in postmenopausal osteoporosis (the DATA-Switch study): extension of a randomised controlled trial. Lancet 2015;386(9999):1147–55.

55. Langdahl BL, Libanati C, Crittenden DB, et al. Romosozumab (sclerostin monoclonal antibody) versus teriparatide in postmenopausal women with osteoporosis transitioning from oral bisphosphonate therapy: a randomised, open-label, phase 3 trial. Lancet 2017;390(10102):1585–94.

56. Lindsay R, Scheele WH, Neer R, et al. Sustained vertebral fracture risk reduction after withdrawal of teriparatide in postmenopausal women with osteoporosis. Arch Intern Med 2004;164(18):2024–30.

57. Cosman F, Lewiecki EM, Ebeling PR, et al. T-Score as an indicator of fracture risk during treatment with romosozumab or alendronate in the ARCH trial. J Bone Miner Res 2020. https://doi.org/10.1002/jbmr.3996.

Update on Rare Adverse Events from Osteoporosis Therapy and Bisphosphonate Drug Holidays

Robert A. Adler, MD[a,b,*]

KEYWORDS

- Osteoporosis • Fracture • Bisphosphonate • Atrial fibrillation • Uveitis
- Osteonecrosis of the jaw • Atypical femoral fracture • Drug holiday

KEY POINTS

- Bisphosphonates remain a first-line agent for osteoporosis and are generally safe and effective.
- Atrial fibrillation and uveitis are rare complications that cannot be predicted.
- Osteonecrosis of the jaw and atypical femoral fracture are also rare and there may be ways to decrease their incidence.
- Most patients can be treated successfully without side effects for 3 to 5 years.
- Each patient must be assessed for drug continuation or holiday at 3 to 5 years.

INTRODUCTION

Osteoporosis remains an important but underappreciated disorder. In the United States, there are at least 2 million osteoporotic fractures every year. Vertebral fractures are the most common, but the most serious fractures, those of the hip (proximal femur), contribute to about one-eighth of the total fractures and a much greater proportion of the morbidity and mortality. It has been estimated that at age 50 women have a 40% to 50% chance of suffering an osteoporotic fracture in their life. For men, the risk is estimated at 13% to 25%. Currently, there is no cure for osteoporosis. All treatments decrease fracture risk, but no treatment eliminates fracture risk. Bisphosphonates remain a first-line treatment for osteoporosis based on their general effectiveness, safety, and relatively low cost. Bisphosphonates decrease vertebral

[a] Endocrinology and Metabolism Section, Central Virginia Veterans Affairs Health Care System, Richmond, VA, USA; [b] Division of Endocrinology, Virginia Commonwealth University, Richmond, VA, USA
* Endocrinology (111P), Central Virginia VA Health Care System, 1201 Broad Rock Boulevard, Richmond, VA 23249.
E-mail address: Robert.adler@va.gov

Endocrinol Metab Clin N Am 50 (2021) 193–203
https://doi.org/10.1016/j.ecl.2021.03.003
0889-8529/21/Published by Elsevier Inc.

fracture risk by 50%. Alendronate (ALN), risedronate, and zoledronic acid (ZA) decrease hip fracture risk by 30% to 40%. For several reasons, patients with osteoporosis are less likely to be diagnosed and treated in 2020 compared with previous years. Well before the novel coronavirus disease-2019 pandemic, diagnosis and treatment were decreasing, and the decrease in medical care for nonviral illness during the pandemic likely decreased diagnosis and treatment rates further. In a review of Medicare data from 2005 to 2015, Lewiecki and colleagues[1] reported that hip fracture in age-adjusted postmenopausal women decreased linearly until 2012, at which point there was no further decrease. In the face of an aging population, fewer women were diagnosed and treated for osteoporosis. In patients who had already suffered an osteoporotic fracture and were at high risk for another, fewer patients are receiving treatment.[2] Despite 2 long-term bisphosphonate treatment studies demonstrating general safety,[3,4] dramatic media reports of serious side effects are the likely cause of a marked decrease in the initiation and persistence of bisphosphonate therapy for osteoporosis.[5] The goal of this article is to provide perspective on how well bisphosphonates work to decrease fracture in relation to how side effects of treatment limit their usefulness and/or lead to treatment discontinuation. A strategy to maximize effectiveness and minimize side effects is provided.

EFFICACY STUDIES AND EFFECT OF DISCONTINUATION

There are 2 widely cited long-term studies of bisphosphonates. In the FLEX study,[3] after about 5 years of ALN, postmenopausal women were randomized to receive 5 more years of ALN or placebo. Hip bone density decreased in the placebo group but remained stable in the active drug group. There were fewer clinical vertebral fractures in those women who received 10 years of ALN compared with the women who received 5 years of ALN followed by a drug holiday (placebo arm) of 5 years. In the HORIZON extension trial,[4] women who had received 3 annual infusions of ZA were randomized to 3 more infusions or 3 placebo infusions. Bone density increased slightly in both groups, but there were fewer morphometric vertebral fractures in the women who had received 6 compared with 3 annual active drug infusions. Interestingly, there were few of the rare side effects that became much more apparent as hundreds of thousands of patients received bisphosphonate treatment. In addition, the studies were too small to detect significant differences in any nonvertebral fracture.

Based on these studies plus supporting post hoc analyses and shorter studies with risedronate and ibandronate, a Task Force of the American Society for Bone and Mineral Research (ASBMR) produced an algorithm for long term osteoporosis treatment.[6] The task force recommended an assessment of fracture risk after 5 years of oral bisphosphonate treatment or after 3 annual infusions of ZA. At that time, if the patient remained at high fracture risk (based on bone density, history of fracture, or other clinical findings), continued treatment was recommended for another 2 to 3 years, when another reassessment was indicated. For patients whose fracture risk was clearly lessened by the first 3 to 5 years of treatment, a drug holiday or interruption was suggested, with reassessment again at 2 to 3 years. After 10 years of treatment, there are no data. Thus, clinical judgment was suggested for management. This general approach to long-term management has been adopted in large part by Guidelines from the American Association of Clinical Endocrinologists[7] and the Endocrine Society,[8] among others. The essential problem is that there are only the 2 major long-term bisphosphonate studies, and it is highly unlikely that there will ever be further randomized controlled trials to supersede or augment them. Observational studies have been helpful to characterize effectiveness and safety, but deficiencies inherent in observational studies prevent more definitive assessments of efficacy and safety.

An approach modified from the ASBMR algorithm is presented elsewhere in this article. It is based on data demonstrating that a single infusion of ZA has an impact on surrogates for fracture for more than 1 year.[9] Studies from New Zealand have shown that bone density increased and then plateaus for at least 2 years after a single infusion of ZA. In addition, bone turnover markers do not return to baseline at 1 year after infusion. In a study[10] of women with osteopenia, although some women had already fractured and could be considered to have osteoporosis based on osteopenia plus a fragility fracture, Reid and colleagues[10] reported that 4 ZA infusions over 6 years led to fewer fractures compared with placebo infusions. In our observational study,[11] men with osteoporosis given ZA had bone resorption markers still suppressed 12, 15, and even 18 months after an infusion. For these reasons and for simplicity and uniformity, this author has recommended[12] that all patients with osteoporosis treated with bisphosphonates undergo an initial 5-year treatment period: 5 years of oral bisphosphonate or 3 ZA infusions spread over 5 years. Although this plan is not supported by specific fracture risk reduction data, it makes clinical sense, and all patients can be instructed that their initial treatment period will be 5 years. As calculated by Black and Rosen,[13] the decrease in osteoporotic fractures far outweighs the incidence of serious side effects during this period. The Common side effects of bisphosphonate treatment section describes the side effects in depth, and then we return to the strategy for longer term management of osteoporosis.

COMMON SIDE EFFECTS OF BISPHOSPHONATE TREATMENT

Much has been written about certain common side effects, such as worsening gastroesophageal reflux or esophageal irritation with oral bisphosphonates. Having gastroesophageal reflux under control before starting a bisphosphonate and keeping the patient in a sitting or upright position during the one-half hour after taking the bisphosphonate with a glass of water decreases these side effects. For those in whom mitigation is not possible, using intravenous bisphosphonate such as ZA or ibandronate is an alternative. However, there is a common side effect of the intravenous bisphosphonates, especially the first time it is given. As many as one-third of patients new to bisphosphonates experience an acute phase reaction after the infusion. This reaction may consist of fever, myalgias, headache, or other flulike symptoms. In most patients it is short lived (24–28 hours) and responsive to antipyretics such as acetaminophen. In perhaps 1% the flulike symptoms are severe enough that the patient goes to a hospital emergency room for relief. Usually after any exposure to bisphosphonates, either previous oral treatment or a previous infusion, the chance of acute phase reaction is markedly decreased. In our own clinics, we encourage good hydration and prophylactic acetaminophen; all patients are informed of the potential side effect.

LESS COMMON SIDE EFFECTS OF BISPHOSPHONATE TREATMENT
Atrial Fibrillation

Four potential side effects merit review: atrial fibrillation, uveitis, osteonecrosis of the jaw (ONJ), and atypical femoral fracture. Although ONJ and atypical femoral fracture have received the most attention in the lay press, it is important to review all four. In the HORIZON registration trial and extension trial, there was an imbalance of atrial fibrillation as a serious adverse event, but not as an overall adverse event. Several observational studies and meta-analyses have tried to clarify whether bisphosphonates, particularly intravenous ZA, is associated with an increased incidence of atrial fibrillation. It was interesting that trials for ZA suggested increased atrial fibrillation, but the hip fracture trial[14] of ZA reported decreased mortality in those patients receiving active drug. An excellent meta-analysis by Kim and colleagues[15] looked at different cardiovascular events (total, atrial fibrillation, myocardial infarction, stroke, and cardiovascular death) in randomized, placebo-controlled trials of oral and intravenous bisphosphonates. The overall conclusion was that bisphosphonates had no beneficial or harmful effects on cardiovascular risk (total and specific types), but there was probably a modest increase in the risk of atrial fibrillation in patients treated with intravenous ZA. A more recent population-based nested case control study from Italy[16] confirmed no increase in cardiovascular risk, but cautioned that patients with osteoporosis are of an age when cardiovascular diseases are common. Thus, finding cardiovascular disease in patients treated for osteoporosis with bisphosphonates should be anticipated.

Inflammatory Eye Disease

There have been a few reports of acute inflammatory eye disease in patients treated with bisphosphonates. From the World Health Organization international pharmacovigilance database,[17] bisphosphonates were the most common drug class associated with drug-induced uveitis, making up more than one-quarter of reported cases. An observational study from Canada[18] compared 10,827 first time bisphosphonate users between 2000 and 2007 with 923,320 nonusers. The relative risk for uveitis was 1.45 (95% confidence interval, 1.25–168) and scleritis 1.51 (95% confidence interval, 1.34–168). The incidence of inflammatory eye disease was reported from a randomized osteoporosis trial in New Zealand.[10,19] In this study, 1054 women receiving ZA were compared with 703 receiving a placebo infusion. In the first group there were 8 cases of acute anterior uveitis and 1 case of episcleritis, whereas there was no inflammatory eye disease in the subjects receiving a placebo infusion. The affected subjects were treated successfully with topical glucocorticoids. In practice, oral glucocorticoids have been used, but it is important to note adequacy of treatment with topical glucocorticoids. The authors suggested that inflammatory eye disease associated with bisphosphonates are likely part of the acute phase reaction widely reported with the first infusion. As potential evidence to support this hypothesis, in another article[20] from the same group, 2 subjects who had acute anterior uveitis from their first infusion underwent rechallenge 18 and 36 months after the first infusion. With careful assessment by ophthalmology before and after the second and third infusions, neither subject developed subjective or objective eye problems.

Osteonecrosis of the Jaw

The first side effect to have a major impact on bisphosphonate initiation and persistence was ONJ. The generally accepted definition of ONJ requires 8 weeks of exposed bone of the mandible or maxilla, despite appropriate therapy. Modern bisphosphonates first came to market in the mid-1990s, and the first reports of ONJ were in 2003. As originally determined by an ASMBR task force[21] and later codified by an international task force,[22] ONJ is defined as exposed bone in the maxillofacial area that remains 8 weeks after clinical assessment in patients exposed to an antiresorptive agent and not related to radiation therapy to the area. Thus, this definition applies to patients with osteoporosis, Paget's disease, and bone disease related to cancer treated with either bisphosphonates or denosumab. For the purpose of this discussion, only patients with osteoporosis are included. It should be noted, however, that most patients with Paget's disease are treated with only 1 infusion of intravenous

ZA and are thus at lower risk for adverse events such as ONJ. In contrast, patients with cancer may receive frequent intravenous bisphosphonate or subcutaneous denosumab treatment and are therefore at much higher risk for ONJ. In patients with osteoporosis, the incidence has generally been estimated as 1 in 10,000 to 100,000 patient-years, and there is some evidence that the incidence increased with the duration of therapy. Many cases were first discovered after an invasive oral procedure such as tooth extraction; this risk factor remains important for ONJ. Poor dental hygiene is considered a risk factor, and some studies have suggested that systemic glucocorticoids and diabetes mellitus may also increase the risk. The pathogenesis of ONJ[23] is considered multifactorial, with suggestions that the antiangiogenic effects of bisphosphonates play a role, as well as infection and suppressed bone turnover.

The lack of a definitive pathogenesis and inadequacy of risk factor assessment implies that only some general suggestions can be made to avoid ONJ in osteoporosis treatment.[24] If patients need invasive dental work at the time of osteoporosis treatment, it is reasonable to get the dental work done and then start bisphosphonate or denosumab. During this time, the nonpharmacologic part of treatment can commence, such as encouraging dietary calcium intake, assessing and enhancing (if needed) vitamin D status, instituting an exercise program, and decreasing fall risk. Then, when the patient has healed from the dental procedures, antiresorptive treatment can begin. All patients need to maximize dental hygiene, although this goal will be challenging for some. The general consensus is that if a patient already on antiresorptive therapy requires invasive dental work, then the antiresorptive treatment should not be stopped. The rationale is that the chance of fracture if the patient is not on treatment far outweighs the chance of ONJ while on treatment. There are 2 other reasons to contemplate. One is that the terminal half-life of bisphosphonates is measured in months or years. Thus, stopping ALN for 2 months before a dental procedure decreases but does not eliminate circulating bisphosphonate in the patient. With denosumab, stopping treatment may lead to rebound vertebral fractures.[25] Despite the low incidence of ONJ and the ability to deal with it in most cases, many patients have not initiated osteoporosis treatment or stopped it because of fear of "their jaw falling off." This fear has led to decreased treatment of osteoporosis.

Atypical Femoral Fractures

Even more worrisome to patients are reports of fractures apparently caused by antiresorptive drugs, leading to further declines in osteoporosis treatment. Taking a fracture prevention medication that may cause a particularly dramatic fracture of the femur has caused great anxiety among patients with osteoporosis. Undoubtedly it has resulted in fewer patients starting or continuing antiresorptive treatment. The updated definition[26] of atypical femoral fractures from an ASBMR Task Force had major and minor features. To be considered an atypical femoral fractures, 4 of 5 major features needed to be present: association with minimal or no trauma, starting at the lateral cortex and being mostly transverse (may become oblique), no or minimal comminution, presence of a medial spike with complete fractures (incomplete would involve lateral cortex only), and the lateral cortex demonstrating a localized reaction ("beaking" or flaring). Minor features include bilaterality (complete or incomplete), prodromal symptom of thigh or groin pain, increased femoral shaft cortex thickness, or delayed fracture healing. None of the minor features were necessary to make the diagnosis. These fractures occur distal to the lesser trochanter and proximal to the supracondylar flare. Typical osteoporotic fractures occur mostly in the neck or trochanteric region of the femur. In the case of an atypical femoral fractures, the patient might be standing or walking normally and fracture, leading to a fall. This sequence contrasts with typical osteoporotic fractures, in which the patient falls and the force of the fall leads to a fracture of the inadequately strong femur.

There are osteoporotic fractures of the femoral shaft as well as the femoral head. An observational study from Italy provides insight into the proportion of fractures that meet criteria for atypical femoral fractures. In this 7-year study[27] there were 4003 femoral fractures, most (3519) of which were in the femoral neck or trochanter region. There were 445 subtrochanteric or shaft fractures, of which 308 were from low or minimal trauma. Only 22 of the 308 met criteria for atypical femoral fractures. It is likely that the majority of the 3519 proximal fractures were osteoporotic, and it is likely that 286 of the shaft fractures were osteoporotic as well. These numbers provide a perspective on the proportions of femoral fractures that could be potentially prevented or caused by antiresorptive agents. Black and Rosen[13] estimated that treating 1000 patients with osteoporosis for 3 years would save 100 osteoporotic fractures for every 1 atypical femoral fractures caused (worst case scenario).

The cause of atypical femoral fractures remains unclear.[28] Although early reports[29] suggested oversuppression of bone turnover, further studies found variable bone turnover status. Atypical femoral fractures resemble stress fractures and some studies (eg, Schilcher et al[30]) have found poor healing within the crack of the fracture, suggesting that the stress of walking prevented healing of the crack. Other studies have suggested that the strain on the lateral cortex is key to atypical femoral fractures. People with anatomy that increases lateral stress seem to be at greater risk for atypical femoral fractures: those with bowing of the femur,[31] varus deformity, or a short angle between the femoral neck and shaft. Interestingly, American women whose ancestors came from some areas of Eastern Asia have an anatomy compatible with lateral femoral cortex strain and in observational studies[32] seem to be at greater risk for atypical femoral fractures. There are anecdotal reports of atypical femoral fractures in younger, active postmenopausal women with osteopenia placed on bisphosphonates to prevent osteoporotic fractures. Such reports provide insights that help to shape an approach to the long-term management of osteoporosis.

APPROACH TO TREAT OSTEOPOROSIS, PREVENT FRACTURES, AND AVOID SIDE EFFECTS

Based on the information presented at the beginning of this article, osteoporotic fracture is common and many can be prevented. What was not mentioned was that hip fractures particularly are deadly. In the elderly (defined for this article as >75 years old), the 1-year mortality from hip fracture is 15% to 30% or more. Of those who survive, about one-half never regain independence. Antiresorptive drugs can prevent hip and other osteoporotic fractures. Bisphosphonates remain first-line treatment for most patients with osteoporosis, and some patients may be treated with denosumab because it may be more potent than bisphosphonates and can be used in patients with declining renal function. In contrast, adverse events after treatment are real, and predicting them, as discussed elsewhere in this article, is difficult. The following approach to osteoporosis treatment is based on the ASBMR Task Force on Long Term Treatment of Osteoporosis.[6] However, this is my personal approach based on the literature plus extensive clinical experience. The goal is to treat those at higher risk for fracture while minimizing side effects.

Nonpharmacologic Management for all Patients at Risk for Osteoporotic Fracture

- Adequate dietary calcium (use supplements only in those with poor dietary intake) and protein

- Adequate vitamin D (supplement to a serum level of 30 ng/mL)
- Weight bearing exercise as tolerated
- Fall risk reduction (eg, avoidance of certain medications and excess alcohol; improving balance, vision, and lower body strength)
- Home safety (eg, night lights, walking aids)
- Discontinue smoking

For Patients at Low Risk for Fracture in the Next 10 Years (Based on History, Physical Exam, Dual Energy X-Ray Absorptiometry, and Fracture Risk Calculators Such as the FRAX)

- All nonpharmacologic methods
- Repeat clinical assessment every 2 years
- Repeat dual energy x-ray absorptiometry (DXA) every 2 to 10 years (depending on the original risk)
- Avoid pharmacologic treatment for osteoporosis

For Patients at Moderate to High Risk of Fracture for the Next 10 Years (Based on the Same Factors)

- If renal function is adequate (estimated creatinine clearance by Cockcroft-Gault formular of >30–35), start ALN 70 mg by mouth weekly or if intolerant of oral bisphosphonates, treat with ZA 5 mg intravenously (slow infusion from 15 to 30 minutes as renal function decreases).
- Oral bisphosphonate-treated patients should be assessed at 3 to 4 months to determine tolerance and adherence.
- For all patients, annual clinical evaluation is recommended to assess adherence to treatment, assessment of new risk factors, encouragement to follow nonpharmacologic recommendations.
- For all patients, DXA assessment at 2 to 3 years may inform clinical conversation about medication adherence and compliance.
- Tell all oral bisphosphonate patients the initial treatment period is 5 years.
- For those on intravenous ZA, give 3 infusions over 5 years (about every 1.5 years) such that their initial treatment period is also 5 years.
- At 5 years, reassess patients clinically and with DXA.

For those with T-scores in spine or hip of less than −2.5, or who have fractured on treatment, or whose FRAX (or other risk calculator) remains high, continue treatment at same dose. For those patients with improvement in bone density, T-score better than of −2.5, and no history of fracture, treatment can be interrupted for 2 to 3 years.

- At 2 to 3 years, reassess patient, including DXA, and use same reasons to discontinue, restart, or continue treatment at same dose. A few patients may need to switch to a different treatment.

For the Highest Risk Patients, Based on Very Low T-Scores, History of Fracture, Frailty, and/or a Very High Risk by a Risk Calculator

- Consider anabolic treatment first: teriparatide or abaloparatide for 1.5 to 2.0 years, or romosozumab for 1 year. Follow this with an antiresorptive and follow the plan for moderate to high-risk patients as discussed elsewhere in this article.

Theis plan keeps those patients who do not need pharmacologic treatment from receiving prescriptions that have potential side effects. Instead, osteoporosis drugs are aimed at those who will benefit most because of their augmented risk for fracture.

Treatment is continued beyond 5 years for those who still need it and interrupted for those who have made real improvements from pharmacologic and nonpharmacologic therapies. For those at the greatest risk, starting with anabolic treatment to increase bone density to a greater degree and improve bone quality is likely to pay dividends in the long run. Whether using anabolic treatment first has an impact on the incidence of side effects from subsequent antiresorptive treatment is not known. What is clear is that it is better to start with an anabolic rather than waiting for the antiresorptive to "fail" before switching to an anabolic drug. A comprehensive program that includes adequate calcium, vitamin D, protein, exercise, fall risk reduction, and careful use of medication should result in the best reduction in fracture while minimizing side effect risk.

Drug Holidays

What happens during the time the previously treated patient interrupts therapy for 2 years or so? As pointed out by Fink and colleagues,[33] the only randomized clinical trial data we have come from the placebo arms of the 2 long-term treatment studies, the 10-year ALN trial (FLEX: 5 years of ALN, then rerandomization to 5 more years of ALN or placebo) and ZA (HORIZON Extension: 3 years of annual ZA infusion rerandomized to 3 more infusions or placebo). In the placebo arm of FLEX, hip bone density decreased and the placebo group had more clinical vertebral fractures than those who continued ALN. In the HORIZON Extension, bone density drifted upward in both groups, but the placebo group had more morphometric vertebral fractures after the 3 placebo infusions compared with those who received the active drug. There are observational studies (eg, Roberts et al[34]) of drug holidays, but such studies have built-in problems of bias: why was one patient picked to stop therapy but another was not? In the case of those patients who stopped treatment on their own, are they any different from those who strictly adhered to treatment? Thus, it is difficult to make conclusions from such studies. There are observational studies (eg, Mignon et al[35]) reporting more fractures in those who discontinued bisphosphonate treatment.

SUMMARY

Many osteoporotic fractures could be prevented by treatment with approved medications, and bisphosphonates remain the most widely used medications based on their efficacy and safety. Nonetheless, fear of side effects contributes to the remarkably low initiation and persistence rates of bisphosphonate drugs for osteoporosis. Identifying those patients at high risk for fracture and mitigating where possible risks for side effects improves the benefits to harms ratio. As a part of a comprehensive program to decrease fracture, careful use of bisphosphonates and other osteoporosis medications can be done safely for the great majority of patients. Recognizing that fracture leads to significant morbidity and mortality, the small risk of side effects must be weighed against the consequences of fracture.

CLINICS CARE POINTS

- All patients at risk for fracture need a comprehensive program of diet, exercise, and fall risk reduction.
- Use nonpharmacologic management and periodic reassessment to manage those at low risk for osteoporotic fracture.

- Bisphosphonates remain a first-line therapy for osteoporosis. This author recommends starting with 5 years of oral ALN or 3 ZA infusions over 5 years.
- Bisphosphonates prevent many fractures compared with rare side effects.
- After 5 years and every 2 to 3 years thereafter, patients need to be assessed for fracture risk. Those remaining at risk should continue treatment, but those who have improved can be considered for a drug holiday.
- Osteoporosis is not cured by treatment. Even those who respond will need continued surveillance.

DISCLOSURE

Research support to institution from Radius Health.

REFERENCES

1. Lewiecki EM, Wright NC, Curtis JR, et al. Hip fracture in the United States, 2002 to 2015. Osteoporos Int 2018;29:717–22.
2. Solomon DH, Johnston SS, Boytsov NN, et al. Osteoporosis medication use after hip fracture in U.S. patients between 2002 and 2011. J Bone Miner Res 2014;29: 1929–37.
3. Black DM, Schwartz AV, Ensrud KE, et al. Effects of continuing or stopping alendronate after 5 years of treatment: the Fracture Intervention Trial Long-term Extension (FLEX): a randomized trial. JAMA 2006;396:2927–38.
4. Black DM, Reid IR, Boonen S, et al. The effects of 3 versus 6 years of zoledronic acid treatment of osteoporosis: a randomized extension of the HORIZON[Pivotal Fracture Trial (PFT). J Bone Miner Res 2012;27:243–54.
5. Jha S, Wang Z, Laucis N, et al. Trends in media reports, oral bisphosphonate prescriptions, and hip fractures 1996-2012: an ecological analysis. J Bone Miner Res 2015;30:2179–87.
6. Adler RA, El-Hajj Fuleihan G, Bauer DC, et al. Managing osteoporosis in patients on long-term bisphosphonate treatment: report of a Task Force of the American Society for Bone and Mineral Research. J Bone Miner Res 2016;31:16–35.
7. Camacho PM, Petak SM, Binkley N, et al. American Association of Clinical Endocrinologists/American College of Endocrinology Clinical Practice Guidelines for the diagnosis and treatment of postmenopausal osteoporosis -2020 update. Endocr Pract 2020;26(Suppl 1):1–46.
8. Eastell R, Rosen CJ, Black DM, et al. Pharmacologic management of Reid osteoporosis in postmenopausal women: an endocrine society clinical practice guideline. J Clin Endocrinol Metab 2019;104:1595–622.
9. Grey A, Bolland MJ, Horne D, et al. Five years of anti-resorptive activity after a single dose of zoledronate: results from a randomized double-blind placebo-controlled trial. Bone 2012;50:1389–93.
10. Reid IR, Horne AM, Mihov B, et al. Fracture prevention with zoledronate in older women with osteopenia. N Engl J Med 2018;379:2407–16.
11. Johnson DA, Williams MI, Petkov VI, et al. Zoledronic acid treatment of osteoporosis: effects in men. Endocr Pract 2010;19:960–7.
12. Adler RA. Duration of anti-resorptive therapy for osteoporosis. Endocrine 2016; 51:222–4.
13. Black DM, Rosen CJ. Clinical practice: postmenopausal osteoporosis. N Engl J Med 2016;374:254–62.

14. Lyles KW, Colon-Emeric CS, Magaziner JS, et al. Zoledronic acid and clinical fractures and mortality after hip fracture. N Engl J Med 2007;357:1799–809.
15. Kim DH, Rogers JR, Fulchino LA, et al. Bisphosphonates and risk of cardiovascular events: a meta-analysis. PLoS One 2015;10:e0122646.
16. Kirchmayer U, Sorge C, Sultana J, et al. Bisphosphonates and cardiovascular risk in elderly patients with previous cardiovascular disease: a population-based nested case-control study in Italy. Ther Adv Drug Saf 2019;10. 20402098619838138.
17. Anquetil C, Salem J-E, Lebrun-Vignes B, et al. Evolving spectrum of drug-induced uveitis at the era of immune checkpoint inhibitors: results from the WHO's pharmacovigilance database. J Autoimmun 2020;111:102454.
18. Etminan M, Forooghian F, Maberley D. Inflammatory ocular adverse events with the use of oral bisphosphonates: a retrospective cohort study. CMAJ 2012;184: E431–4.
19. Patel DV, Bolland M, Nisa Z, et al. Incidence of ocular side effects with intravenous zoledronate: secondary analysis of a randomized controlled trial. Osteoporos Int 2015;26:499–503.
20. Patel DV, Horne A, Mihov B, et al. The effects of re-challenge in patients with a history of acute anterior uveitis following intravenous zoledronate. Calcif Tissue Int 2015;97:58–61.
21. Khosla S, Burr D, Cauley J, et al. Bisphosphonate-associated osteonecrosis of the jaw: report of a Task Force of the American Society for Bone and Mineral Research. J Bone Miner Res 2007;22:1479–91.
22. Khan AA, Morrison A, Hanley DA, et al. Diagnosis and management of osteonecrosis of the jaw: a systematic review and international consensus. J Bone Miner Res 2015;30:3–23.
23. Bejhed RS, Kharazmi M, Halberg P. Identification of risk factors for bisphosphonate-associated atypical femoral fractures and osteonecrosis of the jaw in a pharmacovigilance database. Ann Pharmacother 2016;50:616–24.
24. Hellstein JW, Adler RA, Edwards B, et al. Managing the care of patients receiving antiresorptive therapy for prevention and treatment of osteoporosis. J Am Dent Assoc 2011;142:1243–51.
25. Anastasilakis AD, Poyzos SA, et al. Clinical features of 24 patients with rebound-associated vertebral fractures after denosumab discontinuation: systematic review and additional cases. J Bone Miner Res 2017;32:1291–6.
26. Shane E, Burr D, Abrahamsen B, et al. Atypical subtrochanteric and diaphyseal femoral fractures: second report of a Task Force of the American Society for Bone and Mineral Research. J Bone Miner Res 2014;29:1–23.
27. Pedrazzoni M, Giusti A, Girasole G, et al. Atypical femoral fractures in Italy: a retrospective analysis in a large urban emergency department during a 7-year period (2007-2013). J Bone Miner Metab 2017;35:562–70.
28. Black DM, Abrahamsen B, BouaseinML, et al. Atypical femur fractures: review of epidemiology, relationship to bisphosphonates, prevention, and clinical management. Endocr Rev 2019;40:333–68.
29. Odvina CV, Zerwekh JE, Rao DS, et al. Severely suppressed bone turnover: a potential complication of alendronate therapy. J Clin Endocrinol Metab 2005;90: 1294–301.
30. Schilcher J, Sandberg O, Isaksson H, et al. Histology of 8 atypical femoral fractures: remodeling but no healing. Acta Orthopaedica 2014;85:280–6.
31. Oh Y, Fujita K, Wakabayashi Y, et al. Location of atypical femoral fracture can be determined by tensile stress distribution influenced by femoral bowing and neck-

shaft angle: a CT-based nonlinear finite element analysis model for the assessment of femoral shaft loading stress. Injury 2017;48:2736–43.

32. Lo JC, Hui RI, Grimsrud CD, et al. The association of race/ethnicity and risk of atypical femur fracture among older women receiving oral bisphosphonate therapy. Bone 2016;85:142–7.

33. Fink HA, MacDonald R, Forte ML, et al. Long-term drug therapy and drug discontinuations and holidays for osteoporosis fracture prevention: a systematic review. Ann Intern Med 2019;171:37–50.

34. Roberts J, Castro C, Moore AEB, et al. Changes in bone mineral density and bone turnover in patients on 'drug holiday' following bisphosphonate therapy: real-life clinic setting. Clin Endocrinol 2016;84:509–15.

35. Mignon MA, Taisne N, Legroux I, et al. Bisphosphonate drug holidays in postmenopausal osteoporosis: effect on clinical fracture risk. Osteoporos Int 2017;28:3431–8.

Denosumab Discontinuation in Patients Treated for Low Bone Density and Osteoporosis

Meltem Zeytinoglu, MD, MBA[a],*, Sandra C. Naaman, MD, PhD[b],
Laura T. Dickens, MD[a]

KEYWORDS

- Denosumab • Osteoporosis treatment • Antiresorptive therapy • Bone disorders
- Sequential therapy • Fracture

KEY POINTS

- Denosumab is a potent antiresorptive medication used for the treatment of postmenopausal osteoporosis, osteoporosis in men, glucocorticoid-induced osteoporosis, and to increase bone mass in men at high risk for fracture receiving androgen deprivation therapy for nonmetastatic prostate cancer, and in women at high risk for fracture receiving adjuvant aromatase inhibitor therapy for breast cancer.
- In postmenopausal women with osteoporosis, extended use of denosumab for up to 10 years resulted in progressive increases in bone mineral density and reduced fracture rates, with low rates of associated adverse events.
- Discontinuation of denosumab has been associated with an increased risk for vertebral fractures in some patients.
- In order to prevent rapid bone loss after denosumab discontinuation, it has been recommended that an antiresorptive, especially a bisphosphonate, be used upon discontinuation of denosumab. However, the most effective sequential approach, in terms of which bisphosphonate to use, and at what intervals to be given (intravenous bisphosphonates), following denosumab discontinuation remains unclear.
- Upon transitioning denosumab to a bisphosphonate, close monitoring of ongoing clinical risk, bone turnover markers, and bone mineral density is necessary.

INTRODUCTION

Osteoporosis and low bone density are a chronic disease affecting a significant proportion of older adults.[1,2] In the United States, it has been estimated that there are

[a] Section of Adult and Pediatric Endocrinology, Diabetes, and Metabolism, Department of Medicine, University of Chicago, 5841 South Maryland Avenue, AMB M267, Chicago, IL 60637, USA; [b] Section of General Internal Medicine, Department of Medicine, University of Chicago, 355 East Grand Street, Chicago, IL 60611, USA
* Corresponding author.
E-mail address: mzeytinoglu@uchicago.edu

Endocrinol Metab Clin N Am 50 (2021) 205–222
https://doi.org/10.1016/j.ecl.2021.03.004
0889-8529/21/© 2021 Elsevier Inc. All rights reserved.

more than 2 million osteoporotic fractures per year, many of which result in significant morbidity.[3] Treatments for osteoporosis with substantial efficacy in improving bone mineral density (BMD) and reducing fracture risk are available, and for most patients, the benefits of these treatments significantly outweigh the risk of medication-related adverse effects.[4,5] The most widely used antiresorptive therapies for osteoporosis have been oral and intravenous (IV) bisphosphonates (BSP). The antiresorptive inhibition of osteoclasts occurs primarily when the BSP incorporates into the bony matrix by binding to hydroxyapatite binding sites.[6,7] This integration, within bone surfaces, distinguishes BSP from other more potent osteoporosis therapies by virtue of a residual antiresorptive benefit for a prolonged period after discontinuation. By contrast, the potent antiresorptive effect of denosumab (DMAB) wears off immediately upon treatment discontinuation.

DMAB is a fully humanized monoclonal antibody that binds avidly to the receptor activator of nuclear factor kappa-B ligand (RANKL). The latter is a key precursor to osteoclast differentiation, function, and survival, which in turn regulates bone resorption.[8] States of estrogen deficiency have been shown to increase RANKL exposure to tissues.[9] In part, this explains the significant drop in BMD that is widely observed during the menopausal transition. Blocking RANKL, therefore, has provided an alternative and potent mechanism to attenuate accelerated bone resorption. In addition, neutralizing osteoclast precursors has translated into clinically meaningful suppression of bone remodeling, as demonstrated by change in bone turnover markers (BTM), increases in BMD, and ultimately, reduction in fracture.[4,10–12] DMAB was initially approved for management of postmenopausal osteoporosis (PMO), and its use has subsequently expanded to men with osteoporosis, glucocorticoid-induced osteoporosis, and increasing bone mass in women with breast cancer receiving adjuvant aromatase inhibitor therapy at high risk for fracture, and in men with nonmetastatic prostate cancer receiving androgen deprivation therapy at high risk for fracture.[10,13–16]

EFFICACY OF DENOSUMAB THERAPY

The pivotal 3-year, randomized, double-blinded Fracture Reduction Evaluation of Denosumab in Osteoporosis Every 6 Months (FREEDOM) trial, and its 10-year open-label extension (FREEDOM-Extension), investigated the efficacy of DMAB in mitigating fractures in postmenopausal women as well as its long-term safety and tolerability.[10,12] In the phase 3 FREEDOM trial, 7868 postmenopausal women with osteoporosis were randomized to either 60 mg of DMAB or a placebo administered every 6 months for 3 years.[10] At 36 months, when compared with placebo, women who received DMAB had a relative increase of 9.2% and 6% in BMD of the lumbar spine (LS) and total hip (TH), respectively. Mirroring these densitometric changes in the DMAB group, as compared with placebo, were also improvements in BTM. At months 1, 6, and 36 of the trial, the bone resorption marker C-telopeptide (CTX) levels were significantly suppressed by 86%, 72%, and 72%, respectively. In addition, in the DMAB group, the bone formation marker, procollagen type 1-N terminal propeptide (P1NP) levels were decreased by 18%, 50%, and 76% below the placebo at the same time points. The primary endpoint of the study was new radiographic vertebral fractures, and when compared with placebo, DMAB resulted in a 68% reduction in vertebral fractures. In addition, a 40% reduction in hip fractures and a 20% decrease in nonvertebral fractures were seen.

Given its substantial efficacy in reducing fractures, and the chronicity of osteoporosis, which requires long-term attention and treatment, it was prudent to investigate the long-term safety and tolerability of DMAB, which led to the 10-year FREEDOM-

Extension trial. In this open-label trial, both experimental and control groups who completed the original FREEDOM trial were offered DMAB every 6 months. The outcomes from 5, 6, 8, and 10 years of DMAB exposure were each reported. Remarkably, the results at each of these points demonstrated sustained reductions in BTMs, continued BMD gains, significantly reduced fracture incidence, and consistent safety outcomes.[11,12,17,18] Those who had received DMAB for 10 years experienced persistent gains in the BMD over 10 years, without plateau, with increases of 21.7%, 9.2%, 9%, and 2.7% at the LS, TH, femoral neck (FN), and one-third radius, respectively. Over 7 years of DMAB treatment in the cross-over group (3 years of placebo, followed by 7 years of DMAB), there were BMD gains of 16.5%, 7.4%, 7.1%, and 2.3% at the LS, TH, FN, and one-third radius, respectively. The fracture rate in both groups remained low throughout the study. The 10-year safety data for DMAB demonstrated a low overall rate of adverse events, including serious infection, cellulitis, eczema, and malignancy, and these events did not increase over time. The exposure-adjusted incidences of osteonecrosis of the jaw (ONJ) and atypical femur fracture (AFF) were 5.2 and 0.8 per 10,000 participant-years, respectively.[12]

The robust and sustained gains in BMD, coupled with the relatively low risk for adverse effects and long-term tolerability, make DMAB an attractive option for first-line treatment in osteoporosis management. Indeed, the American Association of Clinical Endocrinologists, in their guidelines on PMO, recommended DMAB as an appropriate initial therapy for most patients at high fracture risk.[19] Several studies have compared DMAB with BSP and demonstrated that DMAB is superior in terms of increasing BMD and in suppression of bone turnover.[14,20,21] In postmenopausal women with osteoporosis, who have been previously treated with oral BSP, DMAB has also shown greater BMD increases and inhibition of bone remodeling than zoledronic acid (ZOL).[22] The DAPS (Denosumab Adherence Preference Satisfaction) study, a randomized crossover study, which enrolled postmenopausal women to receive either 1 year of DMAB or alendronate, followed by alendronate or DMAB in the second year, found that women had greater adherence, compliance, preference, and satisfaction with DMAB as compared with once-weekly alendronate.[23] Among the osteoporosis pharmacotherapies available, other than alendronate, DMAB is unique in terms of having 10-year long-term efficacy and safety data. Therefore, when balancing the risk of osteoporotic fractures with the side-effect profile, especially in those who do not have other risk factors for ONJ or AFF, or high risk for hypocalcemia, and are at higher risk for fracture, the DMAB treatment benefit likely far outweighs the risk of adverse events.

DENOSUMAB DISCONTINUATION: BONE MINERAL DENSITY CHANGES

It is recognized that despite the clear efficacy of DMAB therapy, unlike with the BSP, the therapeutic effect of DMAB is fully reversible upon discontinuation. It was established early on that upon discontinuation of DMAB therapy, there was a transient increase in bone remodeling with associated decline in BMD.[24] At the time of DMAB discontinuation, there is a rapid reversal of RANKL inhibition resulting in increased bone resorption, as evident by a significant increase in BTM. In 2011, Bone and colleagues[24] reported 256 subjects randomized to DMAB or placebo for 24 months (3 injections of DMAB) and then continued off treatment for 24 months with assessment of BMD and BTM at specified time points. With DMAB initiation, there was a rapid decline in BTM, which was sustained during treatment. After 3 months off treatment (9 months from last DMAB dose), CTX increased a median of 63% above baseline and returned to baseline by 18 to 24 months. Bone formation follows a parallel trend, as the same study observed that P1NP increased a median of 47% above baseline after 6 months off treatment (12 months from last DMAB dose). The changes in bone remodeling, reflected by these BTM, have been confirmed by histomorphometric studies.[21,25] Bone histomorphometry from patients treated with DMAB examined at an average of 25.1 months after treatment discontinuation showed normal histology and bone remodeling similar to untreated controls with osteoporosis.[26]

The clinical result of this increase in bone turnover and change in bone remodeling is reflected by changes in BMD. It has been well documented that DMAB discontinuation results in significant bone loss. Several publications observed bone loss in patients after DMAB discontinuation in the FREEDOM and its extension. One study in 2017 examined 12 patients who discontinued DMAB after 7 or 10 years of therapy in the FREEDOM-Extension trial. Eighteen months after the last DMAB dose, subjects were observed to have 9.1% BMD loss at the LS, 12.7% loss at the TH, and 11.0% at the FN. The BMD loss at the TH and FN more than offset prior BMD gains, resulting in an overall decline from baseline before therapy.[27] Another study observed BMD change in 38 women after DMAB discontinuation. At an average of 17 months after the last DMAB dose, there was a mean decline in BMD of 8.1% at the LS, 6.0% at the FN, and 8.4% at the TP. More alarmingly, 5 patients (13.15%) suffered a fragility fracture during that period, including 1 patient with a wrist fracture and 4 patients with vertebral fractures.[28] Notably, it has also been reported that the longer the duration on DMAB, the greater the magnitude of BMD loss measured at all sites, although this has not been consistent across all studies.[27]

DENOSUMAB DISCONTINUATION: FRACTURE RISK

Although it was clear that bone loss occurred upon discontinuation of DMAB, the associated risk for fractures, and more specifically vertebral fractures, was not initially recognized. In 2013, the first analysis of fracture incidence in FREEDOM participants after DMAB was discontinued was published.[26] The study included 797 subjects (470 placebo and 327 DMAB) from the original 36-month FREEDOM trial. Participants had similar baseline characteristics and had received between 2 and 5 doses of DMAB or placebo. At a mean follow-up of 0.8 years after treatment was stopped, the study demonstrated no excess overall fracture risk after discontinuing DMAB, compared with those subjects who had received placebo. Many concluded, then that the transient increase in BTM, and the decline in BMD, did not necessarily translate into clinical fracture risk increase. There was no difference in rates of osteoporosis-related fractures between the DMAB and placebo-treated groups during the off-treatment period of observation. However, it was notable that in this cohort, 28% of patients treated with DMAB were started on another osteoporosis therapy (compared with 42% of placebo). Other limitations of this study include the short period of off-treatment follow-up (median, 0.5 years) and the relatively short duration of DMAB therapy (more than half of patients received 2 or 3 doses). Vertebral fracture risk was not analyzed separately in this study. In addition, more subjects in the placebo treatment groups had a decrease in BMD and fractures during the treatment period, so they were presumably at higher fracture risk at the start of the off-treatment period.

It was not until 2016 that case reports and series began documenting instances of severe spontaneous vertebral fractures after DMAB discontinuation. Aubry-Rozier and colleagues[29] published a report of 3 cases of patients who discontinued DMAB after 5 to 6 doses and developed spontaneous vertebral fractures. One patient had 9 spontaneous fractures 16 months after the last DMAB injection and another suffered 5 spontaneous fractures 10 to 11 months after the last DMAB dose. A larger case series of 24 patients reported 112 vertebral fractures (mean, 4.7 per patient) at 8 to 16 months after last DMAB dose.[30] In this series, one-third of the patients had a history of prevalent vertebral fractures. In 1 case series of 9 women, who received between 2 and 8 doses of DMAB, and in whom 3 had a history of prior vertebral fracture, there were 50 rebound associated vertebral fractures (mean, 5.5 per patient) occurring within 9 to 16 months after DMAB discontinuation.[31] Thus, it became clear there was an urgent need to determine which patients were at highest risk for fractures.

A post hoc analysis of the FREEDOM-Extension trial in 2018 analyzed the risk of new or worsening vertebral fractures in 1001 participants who received DMAB as compared with 470 who received placebo. During the treatment period, risk for vertebral fractures was lower on DMAB therapy compared with placebo (1.2 vs 7.0 per 100 participant-years). After discontinuing therapy with a median follow-up time of 0.5 years (0.2 years for extension), the rate of vertebral fractures in the DMAB-treated group increased to 7.1 per 100 participant-years, which was similar to the rate before (7.0) and after (8.5) discontinuing placebo. Notably, rates of multiple vertebral fractures were higher in patients treated with DMAB (60.7% vs 38.7% in placebo group), and vertebral fracture rates were higher in subjects with prevalent vertebral fractures before treatment.[32]

Two additional features have emerged regarding the incidence of vertebral fractures after DMAB discontinuation. First, there appears to be a risk for ongoing, sequential, rather than single or simultaneous occurrence of multiple fractures.[33,34] Second, that in those who discontinue DMAB compared with those who continue it, the risk for developing multiple vertebral fractures is much greater than the risk for single vertebral fractures. In 1 recent large database of DMAB users, the relative risk of a single vertebral fracture was 4.7 in those who discontinued DMAB versus persistent users, but the risk for multiple vertebral fractures was 14.6 for those discontinuing compared with those with persistent use.[35]

Importantly, the risk of spontaneous vertebral fractures after DMAB therapy is not unique to osteoporosis and has been observed, for example, in women with early-stage breast cancer treated with DMAB to prevent aromatase-inhibitor related bone loss.[36] As the bone community has come to appreciate the scope of this problem, a critical need has arisen for sequential therapeutic strategies to prevent bone loss and vertebral fractures with DMAB discontinuation. When combined, these reports and analyses provided a sufficient weight of evidence to support that, when DMAB is discontinued and no subsequent osteoporosis therapy is given, there is an increased risk of multiple vertebral fractures, and that this risk is greater in those with a history of previous vertebral fractures.

The potential protective effect of prior BSP therapy on subsequent vertebral fracture risk after DMAB discontinuation has been a topic of keen interest. BSP persist in the bone matrix for months or years after treatment is stopped and can provide ongoing protection from bone loss and fractures. A retrospective observational study examined BTM in patients discontinuing DMAB who were previously treated with BSP (n = 17) versus BSP-naive patients (n = 12). Prior BSP treatment duration was for an average of 6.9 years, and the mean time between end of BSP and DMAB initiation was 24.9 months. Median CTX values measured at an average of 11 months after last DMAB injection were significantly higher in the BSP-naive group compared with the prior BSP-treated group, and more subjects in the BSP-naive group had CTX above premenopausal range (9/12%, 75%) compared with the prior BSP-treated group (3/17%, 18%).[37] There are still limited data about the effects of prior BSP use on fracture risk after DMAB discontinuation. In 2019, Bandeira and colleagues[38] reported the case of a woman with postmenopausal osteoporosis, previously treated with alendronate, who experienced multiple severe vertebral fractures within 3 months of a missed dose of DMAB. In addition, a case series in 2018 described 9 high-risk patients who sustained vertebral fractures after DMAB discontinuation and observed that 7 of 9 patients had prior BSP exposure. Six patients had switched directly from BSP to DMAB after an average of 7.4 years of BSP therapy, and the seventh was treated with BSP for 4 years and then teriparatide for 2 years before DMAB. The investigators concluded that among this high-risk cohort, prior BSP use did not appear to have a protective effect.[39] Thus, further research on the effect of pretreatment with BSP is needed.

SEQUENTIAL ANTIRESORPTIVE THERAPY AFTER DENOSUMAB DISCONTINUATION

Given the rebound in bone turnover and bone loss seen after DMAB discontinuation, and the risk of vertebral fractures in some patients discontinuing DMAB, it has been of keen interest to determine the optimal sequential treatment approach for using an antiresorptive after DMAB. An early observational study of 52 patients who received DMAB for 8 years and were observed for 1 year after reported a 6.7% decline in LS and 6.6% decline in TH BMD, but those who took another osteoporosis medication during the study had a smaller decline than those who did not. In addition, of the 8 patients who fractured during the observation period, none received osteoporosis medications before the fracture.[40] To date, few randomized trials have been conducted, and among all data reported, there have been inconsistent results with regard to best treatment approach (eg, oral vs IV BSP), with regard to timing to initiate the antiresorptive after DMAB is discontinued, and on how well BTM correlate with bone loss upon discontinuation of DMAB.

There have been limited reports demonstrating selective estrogen receptor modulators (SERMs) not to be efficacious in the prevention of bone loss after DMAB discontinuation.[41,42] Although further research on this topic may be available in the future, the use of SERMS following DMAB will not be discussed further in this review. Regarding anabolic agents after DMAB, at this time, this approach has not shown any evidence of effectiveness. Notably, whereas the combination of DMAB and teriparatide together resulted in greater increases in spine and hip BMD than either agent alone, teriparatide *after* DMAB actually results in transient bone loss at the spine and hip and progressive bone loss at that radius site.[43,44] In a case report of a 60-year-old woman with a prior history of vertebral fractures, treatment with romosozumab 9 months after DMAB was last given was not able to suppress bone turnover or prevent multiple vertebral fractures.[45] Further observational data on this may be helpful to confirm or clarify the changes in bone turnover and BMD when anabolic agents such as romosozumab or abaloparatide are used after DMAB.

To date, most of the data on antiresorptive use following DMAB have highlighted the role of IV and oral BSP. A few studies have looked at alendronate and ZOL after DMAB and are highlighted in **Table 1**. Several years before it was recognized that DMAB should be followed by another antiresorptive, the DAPS study, a randomized study, evaluated adherence to DMAB and alendronate for 1 year each with a crossover design. Participants were given 12 months of DMAB or alendronate for the first year and then switched to alendronate or DMAB for the second year. BMD remained stable when alendronate was given after DMAB; however, there was a slight increase in BTM.[23] The post hoc analysis of this group was recently published, and it was reported that after 2 doses of DMAB BMD increased by 3% to 6%, and following 1 year of alendronate, BMD increased by 0% to 1%. Although most participants maintained or increased BMD, almost 22% lost BMD at the FN and 16% lost BMD at the

Table 1
Bisphosphonates for prevention of bone loss in patients discontinuing denosumab treatment

Treatment	Patients	BMD	Fractures
ZOL Lehman,[48] 2017 Case series	22 women with PMO 13 pretreated with BSP 9 treatment naive All received 5 DMAB doses followed with single 5-mg dose of ZOL 6 mo after last DMAB	At 24 mo after DMAB discontinued/Zol given, there was loss of BMD gained with DMAB (greater at LS and FN than TH) with no difference between those with prior BSP treatment or treatment naive	At 24 mo after DMAB discontinued, no new vertebral fracture
Reid,[49] 2017 Case series	6 women with PMO All received 14 (7 y) DMAB doses followed by single 5-mg dose of ZOL 6 mo after last DMAB	18–23 mo after DMAB discontinued/ZOL given, significant declines in L-spine and TH BMD	—
Horne,[51,52] 2018, 2019 Retrospective case series	11 women with PMO who completed the FRAME trial (randomized to romosozumab or placebo for 12 mo, followed by DMAB for 2 y). ZOL given at median 65 d (delayed) after trial discontinuation (6 mo and 65 d after last DMAB)	At trial end, LS BMD 17.3% above baseline TH BMD 10.7% above baseline At 1 year later, LS 12.3% above baseline, TH 9.2% above baseline At 2 y later (n = 9), LS 10.2% above baseline, TH 7.6% above baseline	—
Anastasilakis,[55] 2019 Randomized, open-label efficacy study	27 treatment-naive PMO who received single 5 mg ZOL 6 mo after last DMAB (mean, 2.4 y on DMAB before discontinuation)	At 24 mo after DMAB discontinued/ZOL given, L-spine and FN BMD returned to baseline	One patient had a vertebral fracture at 12 mo after ZOL

(continued on next page)

Table 1
(continued)

Treatment	Patients	BMD	Fractures
Ramchand,[64] 2021 Randomized open-label study	53 PMO women who received either standard or high-dose teriparatide with denosumab in the DATA-HD trial for 9 mo. In the extension study, a single 5-mg dose of ZOL was given at month 15 (5–7 mo after last DMAB)	Between months 15 and 27, BMD was maintained in all groups after ZOL infusion. Those who received ZOL early (<26 wk after) had greater decreases in FN (−1.5%) and TH (−3%) BMD. This was not seen at the LS	—
Everts-Graber,[54] 2020 Observational study	120 PMO who received DMAB for 2–5 y (mean, 3 y), followed by single dose of ZOL 6 mo after last DMAB injection	BMD was evaluated 2.5 y after last DMAB (2 y after ZOL) LS decreased by 3.3% (remained +6.4% from baseline before DMAB) TH decreased by 2.2% (remained +2.4% from baseline before DMAB) FN decreased by 1.5% (remained +2.0% from baseline before DMAB)	3 patients had a vertebral fracture (none had multiple fractures) and 4 had nonvertebral fractures
Solling,[56] 2020 Randomized open-label study	61 patients with osteopenia discontinuing DMAB after mean 4.6 y. ZOL was administered 6 (n = 20), 9 (n = 20) mo after the last DMAB, or when BTM increased (n = 21)	At 6 mo after ZOL, LS BMD decreased by 2.1% (6 mo), 4.3% (9 mo), and 3.0% (observed) At 12 mo after ZOL, LS BMD decreased by 4.8% (6 mo), 4.1% (9 mo), and 4.2% (observed) No between group differences	2 women developed incident vertebral fractures
Alendronate Freemantle,[23] 2012 Randomized, crossover DAPS Kendler,[46] 2019 Post hoc analysis	115 PMO women randomized to DMAB for 1 y, followed by alendronate in year 2	From baseline of second year to end of treatment of alendronate, LS 0.6% TH 0.4% FN −0.1%	One humerus fracture in second 12 mo during ALN treatment
Risedronate Horne,[51,52] 2018, 2019	5 women with PMO who completed the FRAME trial	At trial end, LS BMD 17.1% above baseline	—

	(randomized to romosozumab or placebo for 12 mo, followed by DMAB for 2 y). ZOL given at median 8 mo (delayed) after trial discontinuation (6 mo and 65 d after last DMAB)	TH BMD 10.6% above baseline At 1 y later, LS 7.2% above baseline TH 6.7% above baseline At 2 y later (n = 2), TH 6.2% and 8.1% above baseline
Laroche,[65] 2020	18 PMO given 35 mg risedronate per week for 3 mo at 6 mo after last DMAB injection (mean treatment with DMAB 38.7 mo)	At 1 y after DMAB discontinuation, LS whole group −4.6 & Subgroup analysis Treatment naive before DMAB −7.6% Prior BSP exposure −0.3% Prior teriparatide exposure, −6.3% (significantly greater difference between prior BSP exposure and those who were treatment naive or those who received teriparatide prior) TH whole group −1.8% Subgroup analysis Treatment naive before DMAB −4.2% Prior BSP exposure −0.6% Prior teriparatide exposure, −1.5% (significantly greater difference between prior BSP exposure and those who were treatment naive or those who received teriparatide prior)	—

Abbreviation: ALN, alendronate.

LS. It was noted that those who had a greater percentage increase with DMAB lost more BMD after transitioning to alendronate, and this was independent of adherence to alendronate.[46] Two recent case reports of women who were previously treated with BSP and then treated with alendronate after DMAB discontinuation (6–7 doses) and then experienced multiple spontaneous vertebral fractures were published.[47] These fractures occurred at 8 and 12 months after discontinuation.

Several studies have investigated ZOL after DMAB. In 1 retrospective case series published in 2017, 22 women with PMO were given a single dose of ZOL 6 months after the fifth and last DMAB injection. At 24 months after discontinuation of DMAB, there were no vertebral fractures noted, but the single ZOL did not prevent some BMD loss in the L-spine and FN, regardless of whether the patients had received BSP before DMAB treatment.[48] Another series of 6 women who had received 7 years (14 doses) of DMAB therapy, resulting in mean L-spine BMD gain of 18.5% and TH 6.9%, showed that ZOL maintained some, but not all, of these gains.[49] At 18 to 23 months after DMAB was discontinued and ZOL was administered, L-spine BMD remained above pretreatment baseline, but hip did not. The investigators also found that mean P1NP levels in these patients who had received ZOL after DMAB were almost twice as high as postmenopausal women with low bone density who received ZOL without DMAB before. This finding highlighted the possibility that the antiresorptive effect of a single dose of ZOL may be blunted when it is given immediately after DMAB is discontinued. In addition, it was posited that weekly oral BSP, whereby there is more gradual uptake of the BSP as the DMAB-induced suppression of bone turnover wears off, may provide greater protection against bone loss following DMAB discontinuation. One retrospective review of 35 patients who received either an oral (n = 20) or IV BSP (n = 20) after DMAB (mean, 5.6 doses) discontinuation looked at the effect on BMD. Notably, there was a between-group difference in terms of timing between last DMAB and first dose of BSP: 182 days for oral BSP and 275 days for IV ZOL. In this cohort, delaying oral BSP after the last DMAB dose resulted in a greater decline in BMD, whereas delaying IV BSP showed a nonsignificant trend toward preserving or increasing BMD.[50]

There are few studies that have compared the use of different antiresorptives in a similar baseline population. A small case series of women who completed the Fracture Study in Postmenopausal Women with Osteoporosis (FRAME) trial randomized women to 12 months of romosozumab or placebo followed by 24 months of DMAB in all women.[51] In this series, women who completed the trial were offered an oral (risedronate; n = 5) or IV (ZOL; n = 11) BSP after discontinuation of DMAB. Of note in this study was that DMAB was delayed until a median of 65 days (8 months after the last DMAB injection) with the hypothesis that as DMAB wore off, and bone turnover increased, skeletal uptake of the drug might increase and enhance its ability to maintain BMD. The investigators found that administration of ZOL resulted in a 73% retention of treatment effect on LS BMD and an 87% retention of treatment effect on TH BMD. By contrast, the 3 women who did not receive treatment after DMAB was discontinued lost 80% to 90% of the BMD gained during the trial at 12 months after its conclusion. Notably, in the ZOL group, delayed ZOL did suppress the P1NP at 6 months, but it doubled by 12 months, suggesting that a subsequent dose would be needed to maintain BMD gains and that the effect on bone suppression is shorter than in those receiving ZOL without DMAB pretreatment. Interestingly, in a letter published the following year, the investigators reported a 24-month follow-up on BMD from 9 of the 11 patients given ZOL 8 months after DMAB was discontinued.[52] They showed sustained protection against significant bone loss and in suppression of bone resorption, and their study prompts further questions on the timing and frequency of ZOL administration after DMAB discontinuation, and whether BTM can be used to guide treatment timing and frequency. It remains to be answered whether oral versus IV BSP are best to mitigate or prevent bone loss and fractures following DMAB discontinuation. For some patients, the decision may be made by whether they are intolerant to one but not the other.

The use of BTM to guide timing of ZOL was presented last year in a case series of 20 women with postmenopausal osteoporosis, who discontinued DMAB after at least 2 doses.[53] Timing of ZOL was determined by BTM rising above the upper limit of the reference range, which occurred at a mean of 9.4 months after the last DMAB was given. Three months after ZOL was given, median BTM decreased. By 12 months, they returned to levels near those just before ZOL administration, suggesting a recurring rebound. In an observational study of 120 PMO who received a single ZOL upon discontinuation of DMAB (mean, 3 years of use), at 24 months after ZOL, 60% and 49% of the BMD gained by DMAB was maintained at the LS and TH, respectively.[54] During their observation period, 3 individuals had single vertebral fractures, and 4 individuals had nonvertebral fractures. Several notable findings were that there was no association between loss of BMD and prior treatment with antiresorptive treatments, history of prevalent fractures, or greater BMD gains from DMAB (>9% at LS). BMD decrease after DMAB did not correlate with BMD gained during DMAB.

Two randomized clinical trials have assessed BMD changes following ZOL administration. Anastasilakis and colleagues[55] conducted a prospective randomized clinical trial of ZOL for the prevention of bone loss in women discontinuing DMAB. Fifty-seven women with no treatment before DMAB were randomized to receive either a single ZOL infusion 6 months after the last DMAB dose (n = 27; mean time on DMAB 2.4 years) or 2 additional DMAB doses, followed by observation with no additional treatment for 12 months after the last DMAB (n = 30; mean time on DMAB before the trial 2 years). In those who received ZOL, at 24 months after ZOL, L-spine and FN BMD returned to baseline, but in the women who received 2 more DMAB doses, and then were observed for 12 months after the last dose, BMD decreased significantly by a mean of 4.82% at 12 months after the last DMAB dose was given. These values were significantly lower than baseline. The difference in change in BMD between the ZOL and DMAB groups was also statistically significant. A similar observation was made for a secondary outcome of FN BMD. BTM were also assessed. In the ZOL group, there was a small but significant increase in BTM P1NP and CTX during the first 12 months after ZOL was given with stabilization thereafter. In the DMAB group, 3 months after the last DMAB was given (at 15 months), BTM increased significantly and remained elevated at 24 months. Notably, BTM were not associated with BMD changes in either group. In this study, delayed ZOL was able to prevent bone loss for at least 2 years after DMAB was discontinued, and this was independent of the rate of bone turnover, that is, even when considering baseline BTM, BTM could not predict the rate of bone loss here. Of note, however, among the 27 patients who received ZOL, there was variability in individual responses to ZOL in terms of preventing bone loss with 3 and 4 women actually having had significant decline in LS or FN BMD, respectively. Sølling and colleagues[56] published the results of a randomized trial whereby 61 postmenopausal women and men over the age of 50 years (mean age, 68 years) with osteopenia, who had received DMAB for at least 2 years (mean, 4.6 years), were randomized to receive a single infusion of ZOL at 6 months or 9 months after last DMAB or when BTM increased after the last DMAB injection. In all 3 groups, there was significant reduction in BMD at the LS, TH, and FN with some patients in all groups achieving losses greater than the least significant change. Thus, at 12 months, a single infusion of ZOL was not enough to completely prevent bone loss regardless of when it was given nor was it able to maintain suppression of bone turnover, although in the 6-month group, CTX did initially decrease, followed by a rapid increase. They concluded then that the initial decline in bone turnover makes 6 months the most likely optimal time for initial ZOL infusion, but also that given the rapid increase in bone turnover after initial suppression despite the initial ZOL, bone turnover should be monitored, perhaps at 3 and 6 months, to see if a second infusion of ZOL is needed if BTM increases rapidly and that further investigation in this is needed.

WHEN SHOULD DENOSUMAB BE DISCONTINUED?

In the absence of a reversible secondary cause, or a curative treatment, low BMD and osteoporosis are a chronic disease necessitating continued follow-up, monitoring, and treatment. A historical benefit of the BSP has been their prolonged suppression of bone resorption for up to several years after discontinuation. Albeit more potent than BSP, novel osteoporosis therapies, including the anabolic therapies teriparatide and abaloparatide, and the dual-action anabolic and antiresorptive romosozumab, as well as DMAB, are all characterized by rapid reversal of effect upon discontinuation, thus, the need to follow these therapies with another antiresorptive in order to maintain at least some of the gains observed on these medications. Despite the low risk of adverse events seen with DMAB, there are no data on safety and efficacy beyond 10 years. For those with osteoporosis at lower- or intermediate-fracture risk, 10 years may be longer than needed to achieve therapeutic goals, and in these patients, discontinuing therapy may help to eliminate any risk of adverse events.

There is no clear consensus for optimal duration of therapy, which should be individualized to the patient based on several factors, including BMD T-score at the start of and during therapy, history of prior and recent fractures, risk factors, such as other medications or medical conditions that may contribute to ongoing bone loss, age, and overall fragility, and fall risk. Although the most important factors in the therapeutic decision are reduction of future fracture risk and risk of adverse events, BMD has been described as the most useful clinical target to follow. Some groups have emphasized a "treat-to-target" approach for BMD, whereby therapy should be continued at least until a threshold BMD T-score is met, such as a hip T-score of greater than −2.5 or greater than 2.0. The Fracture Intervention Trial Long-term Extension (FLEX) study of long-term use of alendronate (10 years) and the Health Outcomes and Reduced Incidence with Zoledronic Once Yearly (HORIZON) Pivotal Fracture Trial, where ZOL was given for 6 annual infusions, demonstrated that a low hip T-score between −2 and −2.5 (FLEX) and less than −2.5 (HORIZON) predicted an advantageous response to continued therapy.[57,58] Using these data, the American Society for Bone and Mineral Research (ASBMR) Task Force issued a report on managing osteoporosis in patients on long-term BSP, whereby a hip T-score of less than −2.5 or other high-risk criteria, including clinical risk factors, such as age and fractures, or a Fracture Risk Assessment (FRAX) tool score for 10-year risk of major osteoporotic fracture or hip fracture of greater than 20% or 3%, respectively, favored continued treatment.[59] The ASBMR and National Osteoporosis Foundation also published a collaborative report from their Working Group on Goal-Directed Treatment on Osteoporosis, whereby the goals of treatment should be when there is a hip T-score of greater than −2.5, freedom from fracture, or an FRAX risk below the threshold for initiating treatment.[60] Most recently, a consensus panel of European experts concluded that although the primary goals are to reduce fracture risk and recover prefracture functional level in those with fractures, hip BMD does appear to be the most appropriate target for a treat-to-target approach.[61] Recent guidelines from the Endocrine Society, American Association of Clinical Endocrinologists, and the European Calcified Tissue Society all acknowledge the potential therapeutic benefits of DMAB, but also highlight the risk of adverse effects with DMAB discontinuation, which make careful selection of the patient to initiate DMAB of the utmost importance.[4,62,63]

APPROACH TO DENOSUMAB DISCONTINUATION

To date, the reports of fractures occurring following DMAB discontinuation have been almost exclusively related to vertebral fractures. At this time, although the precise approach for using a BSP upon discontinuing DMAB is still under investigation, the weight of evidence supports that in most patients, BSP will at least mitigate the rapid loss of BMD and reduce fractures compared with discontinuation alone. Therefore, in most cases, it would not be ethical to continue to observe patients without any intervention following discontinuation of DMAB, in order to monitor long term for any other excess risk attributable to DMAB discontinuation. Continued retrospective analyses may help for other sites, and randomized trials will help clarify some of the questions that remain. At this time, several features, highlighted in the Clinics Care Points, have emerged with regard to BMD loss and fracture risk after DMAB discontinuation.

Until further studies highlighting best practices for DMAB use and discontinuation in patients with low bone density and osteoporosis are available, the authors recommend that in a younger postmenopausal or younger male patient, if another therapy with similar or greater efficacy is not contraindicated, DMAB should not be used. In younger patients with contraindications to other therapies, or in whom there is renal insufficiency (with extra attention to avoid treatment-related hypocalcemia), DMAB may still be considered. When possible, especially in patients with a history of prior vertebral fractures, an anabolic therapy, such as abaloparatide, teriparatide, or romosozumab, should be used before, but not immediately after DMAB therapy, unless the patient is expected to be able to stay on DMAB indefinitely (eg, when life expectancy is not near or >10 years). When DMAB is initiated, and during therapy, patients should be counseled on the importance of not delaying therapy after 6 months or missing doses. Upon discontinuation of DMAB, a vertebral fracture assessment by DXA should be considered along with BMD to assess for posttreatment baseline vertebral fractures. Alendronate or ZOL should be initiated without delay (at 6 months after the last DMAB dose). If possible, baseline BTM should be monitored at the time of starting BSP and followed at 1, 3, 6, and 12 months. If the patient experiences a fracture, their CTX doubles from nadir or increases to $\geq$300 pg/mL, or there is a loss of BMD of greater than 5% at the LS or TH, the authors recommend stopping the BSP and resuming DMAB until additional sequential therapy approaches are available.

SUMMARY

In conclusion, DMAB is a potent antiresorptive osteoporosis therapy that is generally well tolerated and associated with low risk of adverse effects. Over 10 years, DMAB therapy results in progressive BMD gains and consistent fracture risk reduction without an increase in adverse events. Nevertheless, upon discontinuation, there is a rapid increase in bone turnover and loss of BMD, and an increased risk of multiple vertebral fractures, especially in those with prior history of vertebral fractures. Upon discontinuation of DMAB, alendronate or ZOL should be given without delay, and the patient should be monitored closely for evidence of ongoing increase in bone turnover, significant loss of BMD, or new fractures.

CLINICS CARE POINTS

Established or likely factors of BMD loss and fracture risk after denosumab is discontinued

- Denosumab discontinuation, especially when not followed by a bisphosphonate, is associated with an increased risk of multiple vertebral fractures.
- Risk of vertebral fractures in those who discontinue denosumab is even greater in those with a history of prior vertebral fractures.
- Larger gains in BMD during denosumab treatment are associated with greater loss of BMD when treatment is discontinued.
- Both oral (alendronate) and intravenous (zoledronic acid) bisphosphonates after denosumab preserve some, but not all, of the BMD gained with denosumab.
- Fractures have been reported soon after denosumab is discontinued, therefore bisphosphonates should be initiated without delay.

Areas where further research is needed

- Treatment with a bisphosphonate before denosumab may or may not result in greater preservation of BMD when denosumab is discontinued.
- Bone turnover markers, likely, but not consistently, correlate with BMD change following denosumab discontinuation.
- Whether longer duration of treatment with denosumab is associated with greater loss of BMD.
- Whether oral or intravenous bisphosphonates are most effective in preserving BMD and reducing fracture risk after denosumab.
- Duration of bisphosphonate treatment needed after denosumab is discontinued, and for zoledronic acid, the frequency needed to mitigate increases in bone turnover and prevent loss of BMD.

DISCLOSURE

M. Zeytinoglu, L. Dickens, and S. Naaman have no disclosures to report.

REFERENCES

1. Looker A, Frenk S. Percentage of adults aged 65 and over with osteoporosis or low bone mass at the femur neck or lumbar spine: United States, 2005–2010. Division of Health and Nutrition Examination Surveys. Centre for Disease Control and Prevention; 2015.
2. Wright NC, Looker AC, Saag KG, et al. The recent prevalence of osteoporosis and low bone mass in the United States based on bone mineral density at the femoral neck or lumbar spine. J Bone Mineral Res 2014;29(11):2520–6.
3. Hansen D, Bazell C, Pelizzari P, et al. Milliman Research Report: Medicare cost of osteoporotic fractures. The Clinical and Cost Burden of an Important Consequence of Osteoporosis. National Osteoporosis Foundation. Milliman Inc.; 2019. p. 14–6.
4. Eastell R, Rosen CJ, Black DM, et al. Pharmacological management of osteoporosis in postmenopausal women: an Endocrine Society Clinical Practice Guideline. J Clin Endocrinol Metab 2019;104(5):1595–622.
5. Black DM, Rosen CJ. Postmenopausal osteoporosis. N Engl J Med 2016;374(3):254–62.

6. Nancollas G, Tang R, Phipps R, et al. Novel insights into actions of bisphospho-nates on bone: differences in interactions with hydroxyapatite. Bone 2006;38(5): 617–27.
7. McClung M, Harris ST, Miller PD, et al. Bisphosphonate therapy for osteoporosis: benefits, risks, and drug holiday. Am J Med 2013;126(1):13–20.
8. Vega D, Maalouf NM, Sakhaee K. The role of receptor activator of nuclear factor-κB (RANK)/RANK ligand/osteoprotegerin: clinical implications. J Clin Endocrinol Metab 2007;92(12):4514–21.
9. Eghbali-Fatourechi G, Khosla S, Sanyal A, et al. Role of RANK ligand in mediating increased bone resorption in early postmenopausal women. J Clin Invest 2003; 111(8):1221–30.
10. Cummings SR, Martin JS, McClung MR, et al. Denosumab for prevention of frac-tures in postmenopausal women with osteoporosis. N Engl J Med 2009;361(8): 756–65.
11. Papapoulos S, Lippuner K, Roux C, et al. The effect of 8 or 5 years of denosumab treatment in postmenopausal women with osteoporosis: results from the FREEDOM Extension study. Osteoporos Int 2015;26(12):2773–83.
12. Bone HG, Wagman RB, Brandi ML, et al. 10 years of denosumab treatment in postmenopausal women with osteoporosis: results from the phase 3 randomised FREEDOM trial and open-label extension. Lancet Diabetes Endocrinol 2017;5(7): 513–23.
13. Orwoll E, Teglbjærg CS, Langdahl BL, et al. A randomized, placebo-controlled study of the effects of denosumab for the treatment of men with low bone mineral density. J Clin Endocrinol Metab 2012;97(9):3161–9.
14. Saag KG, Wagman RB, Geusens P, et al. Denosumab versus risedronate in glucocorticoid-induced osteoporosis: a multicentre, randomised, double-blind, active-controlled, double-dummy, non-inferiority study. Lancet Diabetes Endocri-nol 2018;6(6):445–54.
15. Ellis GK, Bone HG, Chlebowski R, et al. Randomized trial of denosumab in pa-tients receiving adjuvant aromatase inhibitors for nonmetastatic breast cancer. J Clin Oncol 2008;26(30):4875–82.
16. Smith MR, Egerdie B, Toriz NH, et al. Denosumab in men receiving androgen-deprivation therapy for prostate cancer. N Engl J Med 2009;361(8):745–55.
17. Bone HG, Chapurlat R, Brandi M-L, et al. The effect of three or six years of deno-sumab exposure in women with postmenopausal osteoporosis: results from the FREEDOM extension. J Clin Endocrinol Metab 2013;98(11):4483–92.
18. Papapoulos S, Chapurlat R, Libanati C, et al. Five years of denosumab exposure in women with postmenopausal osteoporosis: results from the first two years of the FREEDOM extension. J Bone Mineral Res 2012;27(3):694–701.
19. Camacho PM, Petak SM, Binkley N, et al. American Association of Clinical Endo-crinologists/American College of Endocrinology clinical practice guidelines for the diagnosis and treatment of postmenopausal osteoporosis—2020 update. En-docr Pract 2020;26(s1):1–46.
20. Roux C, Hofbauer L, Ho P, et al. Denosumab compared with risedronate in post-menopausal women suboptimally adherent to alendronate therapy: efficacy and safety results from a randomized open-label study. Bone 2014;58:48–54.
21. Brown J, Roux C, Ho P, et al. Denosumab significantly increases bone mineral density and reduces bone turnover compared with monthly oral ibandronate and risedronate in postmenopausal women who remained at higher risk for frac-ture despite previous suboptimal treatment with an oral bisphosphonate. Osteo-poros Int 2014;25(7):1953–61.

22. Miller P, Pannacciulli N, Brown J, et al. Denosumab or zoledronic acid in postmenopausal women with osteoporosis previously treated with oral bisphosphonates. J Clin Endocrinol Metab 2016;101(8):3163–70.

23. Freemantle N, Satram-Hoang S, Tang E-T, et al. Final results of the DAPS (Denosumab Adherence Preference Satisfaction) study: a 24-month, randomized, crossover comparison with alendronate in postmenopausal women. Osteoporos Int 2012;23(1):317–26.

24. Bone HG, Bolognese MA, Yuen CK, et al. Effects of denosumab treatment and discontinuation on bone mineral density and bone turnover markers in postmenopausal women with low bone mass. J Clin Endocrinol Metab 2011;96(4):972–80.

25. Brown JP, Dempster DW, Ding B, et al. Bone remodeling in postmenopausal women who discontinued denosumab treatment: off-treatment biopsy study. J Bone Mineral Res 2011;26(11):2737–44.

26. Brown JP, Roux C, Törring O, et al. Discontinuation of denosumab and associated fracture incidence: analysis from the Fracture Reduction Evaluation of Denosumab in Osteoporosis Every 6 Months (FREEDOM) trial. J Bone Mineral Res 2013;28(4):746–52.

27. Popp AW, Varathan N, Buffat H, et al. Bone mineral density changes after 1 year of denosumab discontinuation in postmenopausal women with long-term denosumab treatment for osteoporosis. Calcified Tissue Int 2018;103(1):50–4.

28. Zanchetta M, Boailchuk J, Massari F, et al. Significant bone loss after stopping long-term denosumab treatment: a post FREEDOM study. Osteoporos Int 2018; 29(1):41–7.

29. Aubry-Rozier B, Gonzalez-Rodriguez E, Stoll D, et al. Severe spontaneous vertebral fractures after denosumab discontinuation: three case reports. Osteoporos Int 2016;27(5):1923–5.

30. Anastasilakis AD, Polyzos SA, Makras P, et al. Clinical features of 24 patients with rebound-associated vertebral fractures after denosumab discontinuation: systematic review and additional cases. J Bone Mineral Res 2017;32(6):1291–6.

31. Lamy O, Gonzalez-Rodriguez E, Stoll D, et al. Severe rebound-associated vertebral fractures after denosumab discontinuation: 9 clinical cases report. J Clin Endocrinol Metab 2017;102(2):354–8.

32. Cummings SR, Ferrari S, Eastell R, et al. Vertebral fractures after discontinuation of denosumab: a post hoc analysis of the randomized placebo-controlled FREEDOM trial and its extension. J Bone Mineral Res 2018;33(2):190–8.

33. Anastasilakis AD, Evangelatos G, Makras P, et al. Rebound-associated vertebral fractures may occur in sequential time points following denosumab discontinuation: need for prompt treatment re-initiation. Bone Rep 2020;12:100267.

34. Niimi R, Kono T, Nishihara A, et al. Second rebound-associated vertebral fractures after denosumab discontinuation. Arch Osteoporos 2020;15(1):7.

35. Tripto-Shkolnik L, Fund N, Rouach V, et al. Fracture incidence after denosumab discontinuation: real-world data from a large healthcare provider. Bone 2020; 130:115150.

36. Gonzalez-Rodriguez E, Aubry-Rozier B, Stoll D, et al. Sixty spontaneous vertebral fractures after denosumab discontinuation in 15 women with early-stage breast cancer under aromatase inhibitors. Breast Cancer Res Treat 2020;179(1):153–9.

37. Uebelhart B, Rizzoli R, Ferrari SL. Retrospective evaluation of serum CTX levels after denosumab discontinuation in patients with or without prior exposure to bisphosphonates. Osteoporos Int 2017;28(9):2701–5.

38. Bandeira F, Torres G, Bandeira E, et al. Multiple severe vertebral fractures during the 3-month period following a missed dose of denosumab in a postmenopausal

woman with osteoporosis previously treated with alendronate. Int J Clin Pharmacol Ther 2019;57(3):163.

39. Tripto-Shkolnik L, Rouach V, Marcus Y, et al. Vertebral fractures following denosumab discontinuation in patients with prolonged exposure to bisphosphonates. Calcified Tissue Int 2018;103(1):44–9.

40. McClung M, Wagman RB, Miller P, et al. Observations following discontinuation of long-term denosumab therapy. Osteoporos Int 2017;28(5):1723–32.

41. Gonzalez-Rodriguez E, Stoll D, Lamy O. Raloxifene has no efficacy in reducing the high bone turnover and the risk of spontaneous vertebral fractures after denosumab discontinuation. Case Rep Rheumatol 2018;2018:5432751.

42. Ebina K, Miyama A, Hirao M, et al. Assessment of the effects of sequential treatment after discontinuing denosumab in 64 patients with postmenopausal osteoporosis. Abstract presented at: American Society of Bone and Mineral Research, Orlando, FL, 2019.

43. Tsai JN, Uihlein AV, Lee H, et al. Teriparatide and denosumab, alone or combined, in women with postmenopausal osteoporosis: the DATA study randomised trial. Lancet 2013;382(9886):50–6.

44. Leder BZ, Tsai JN, Uihlein AV, et al. Denosumab and teriparatide transitions in postmenopausal osteoporosis (the DATA-Switch study): extension of a randomised controlled trial. Lancet 2015;386(9999):1147–55.

45. Kashii M, Ebina K, Kitaguchi K, et al. Romosozumab was not effective in preventing multiple spontaneous clinical vertebral fractures after denosumab discontinuation: a case report. Bone Rep 2020;13:100288.

46. Kendler D, Chines A, Clark P, et al. Bone mineral density after transitioning from denosumab to alendronate. J Clin Endocrinol Metab 2019;105(3):e255–64.

47. Lamy O, Fernández-Fernández E, Monjo-Henry I, et al. Alendronate after denosumab discontinuation in women previously exposed to bisphosphonates was not effective in preventing the risk of spontaneous multiple vertebral fractures: two case reports. Osteoporos Int 2019;30(5):1111–5.

48. Lehmann T, Aeberli D. Possible protective effect of switching from denosumab to zoledronic acid on vertebral fractures. Osteoporos Int 2017;28(10):3067–8.

49. Reid IR, Horne AM, Mihov B, et al. Bone loss after denosumab: only partial protection with zoledronate. Calcified Tissue Int 2017;101(4):371–4.

50. Dickens L, Vokes T. Oral vs intravenous bisphosphonates for preventing bone loss after denosumab discontinuation. Abstract presented at: American Society of Bone and Mineral Research, Orlando, FL, 2019.

51. Horne AM, Mihov B, Reid IR. Bone loss after romosozumab/denosumab: effects of bisphosphonates. Calcified Tissue Int 2018;103(1):55–61.

52. Horne AM, Mihov B, Reid IR. Effect of zoledronate on bone loss after romosozumab/denosumab: 2-year follow-up. Calcified Tissue Int 2019;105(1):107–8.

53. Popp A, Bock O, Senn C, et al. Early recurrence of increased bone turnover markers after initial response to single dose zoledronate following denosumab discontinuation in postmenopausal women. Abstract presented at: American Society of Bone and Mineral Research, Orlando, FL, 2019.

54. Everts-Graber J, Reichenbach S, Ziswiler HR, et al. A single infusion of zoledronate in postmenopausal women following denosumab discontinuation results in partial conservation of bone mass gains. J Bone Mineral Res 2020;35(7):1207–15.

55. Anastasilakis AD, Papapoulos SE, Polyzos SA, et al. Zoledronate for the prevention of bone loss in women discontinuing denosumab treatment. A prospective 2-year clinical trial. J Bone Miner Res 2019;34(12):2220–8.

56. Sølling AS, Harsløf T, Langdahl B. Treatment with zoledronate subsequent to de-nosumab in osteoporosis: a randomized trial. J Bone Miner Res 2020;35(10): 1858–70.

57. Black DM, Schwartz AV, Ensrud KE, et al. Effects of continuing or stopping alendronate after 5 years of treatment: the Fracture Intervention Trial Long-term Extension (FLEX): a randomized trial. JAMA 2006;296(24):2927–38.

58. Black DM, Reid IR, Boonen S, et al. The effect of 3 versus 6 years of zoledronic acid treatment of osteoporosis: a randomized extension to the HORIZON-Pivotal Fracture Trial (PFT). J Bone Mineral Res 2012;27(2):243–54.

59. Adler RA, El-Hajj Fuleihan G, Bauer DC, et al. Managing osteoporosis in patients on long-term bisphosphonate treatment: report of a task force of the American Society for Bone and Mineral Research. J Bone Mineral Res 2016;31(1):16–35.

60. Cummings SR, Cosman F, Lewiecki EM, et al. Goal-directed treatment for osteo-porosis: a progress report from the ASBMR-NOF working group on goal-directed treatment for osteoporosis. J Bone Mineral Res 2017;32(1):3–10.

61. Thomas T, Casado E, Geusens P, et al. Is a treat-to-target strategy in osteoporosis applicable in clinical practice? Consensus among a panel of European experts. Osteoporos Int 2020;31(12):2303–11.

62. Camacho PM, Petak SM, Binkley N, et al. American Association of Clinical Endo-crinologists and American College of Endocrinology clinical practice guidelines for the diagnosis and treatment of postmenopausal osteoporosis—2016. Endocr Pract 2016;22(s4):1–42.

63. Tsourdi E, Zillikens MC, Meier C, et al. Fracture risk and management of discon-tinuation of denosumab therapy: a systematic review and position statement by ECTS. J Clin Endocrinol Metab 2020.

64. Ramchand SK, David NL, Lee H, et al. Efficacy of Zoledronic Acid in Maintaining Areal and Volumetric Bone Density After Combined Denosumab and Teriparatide Administration: DATA-HD Study Extension. Journal of Bone and Mineral Research 2021.

65. Laroche M, Couture G, Ruyssen-Witrand A, et al. Effect of risedronate on bone loss at discontinuation of denosumab. Bone Reports 2020;13:100290.

Role of Bone Turnover Markers in Osteoporosis Therapy

Sumeet Jain, MD

KEYWORDS

- Bone turnover markers • Osteoporosis • CTX • PINP • Bisphosphonate holiday
- Secondary osteoporosis • Adherence

KEY POINTS

- Familiarize yourself with the variables that affect bone turnover marker variability.
- Learn how bone turnover markers are affected by secondary causes of osteoporosis.
- Interpret bone turnover markers with an understanding of least significant change and statistical significance.
- Use bone turnover markers for rapid feedback on therapeutic interventions.

INTRODUCTION

Osteoporotic fractures are a growing public health problem with an aging global population. One in 3 women and 1 in 5 men over the age of 50 will suffer an osteoporotic fracture in their lifetime.[1] Osteoporosis causes significant morbidity and mortality and is expected to cost $25 billion per year just in the United States by 2025.[2] The annual incidence of hip fractures in Asia is expected to more than double by 2050, when a projected 50% of worldwide hip fractures will occur in Asia.[3] Screening for osteoporosis and comprehensive recurrent fracture prevention is underperformed and undervalued. Bone turnover markers have a growing role in osteoporosis management, and strong clinical interest exists for the use of bone turnover markers as part of the comprehensive evaluation and treatment of osteoporosis.

DEFINITION

Bone turnover markers are noninvasive blood or urine biomarkers used to dynamically evaluate bone remodeling. Bone remodeling is a constant process that repairs microfractures in bones by coupling bone resorption to bone formation. Osteoclasts release

Division of Endocrinology and Metabolism, Department of Medicine, Rush University Medical Center, 1725 West Harrison Street, Suite 250, Chicago, IL 60612, USA
E-mail address: Sumeet_Jain@rush.edu

Endocrinol Metab Clin N Am 50 (2021) 223–237
https://doi.org/10.1016/j.ecl.2021.03.007
0889-8529/21/© 2021 Elsevier Inc. All rights reserved.

catabolized bone proteins into the blood that can be measured to estimate bone resorption. Osteoblasts form the osteoid framework of bones and secrete protein byproducts into the blood that can be measured to estimate bone formation.

DUAL-ENERGY X-RAY ABSORPTIOMETRY DXA SCAN LIMITATIONS

Dual-energy X-ray absorptiometry (DXA) scans, our most used screening tool for osteoporosis, find a high-risk cohort for fracture that are clear candidates for fracture reducing therapy, but are still lacking for ideal clinical use. Bone density in the osteoporotic range on a DXA scan does not capture over half of women who go on to fracture.[4] Impairments in bone quality are often not captured in bone density measurements. Just as concerning, when people have devastating osteoporotic fractures, treatment and workup to prevent recurrent fracture too frequently never occur despite a 10% risk of recurrent fracture within 1 year and 31% risk of recurrent fracture within 5 years.[5] In the already inadequate subset of people with osteoporosis who receive treatment, secondary osteoporosis evaluation is commonly not performed despite 20% to 30% of postmenopausal women and 50% of men with osteoporosis having a secondary cause of osteoporosis.[6] Even after therapeutic intervention is made, it can take 1 to 2 years to confirm stability or improvement on a DXA scan. Delays in monitoring response to therapy contribute to high rates of self-discontinuation of osteoporosis treatments that are reported to be as high as 30% to 60% and are associated with more fractures and higher cost.[7,8]

ROLE OF BONE TURNOVER MARKERS

When bone turnover markers are used with a thorough understanding of their flaws and limitations, they help fill these gaps in clinical osteoporosis management by expediting feedback in response to therapy for clinicians, providing positive reinforcement on treatment adherence for patients with a silent disease, enhancing fracture prediction modestly, and demonstrating imbalances in bone resorption and bone formation that increase clinical suspicion for secondary causes of osteoporosis. These problems are not just academic and are being increasingly recognized by clinicians, as filling clinical needs as demonstrated by a doubling of bone turnover marker testing in real-world US insurance claims data between 2008 and 2018.[9]

STANDARDIZED BONE TURNOVER MARKERS ARE N-TERMINAL PROPEPTIDE OF TYPE I COLLAGEN AND C-TERMINAL TELOPEPTIDE OF TYPE I COLLAGEN

N-terminal propeptide of type I collagen (PINP) is the recommended standard biochemical marker of bone formation, and C-terminal telopeptide of type I collagen (CTX) is the recommended standard biochemical marker of bone resorption.

Historically, there was a lack of standardization for which bone turnover markers should be used in both clinical and research settings, which greatly impaired external validity of bone turnover marker studies. The lack of standardized reference bone turnover markers was addressed by the International Osteoporosis Foundation (IOF) and the International Federation of Clinical Chemistry (IFCC) in 2010 when they chose PINP and CTX as preferred biomarkers of bone formation and bone resorption.[10] In the subsequent decade, the clinical usefulness of bone turnover markers has greatly improved. Reference ranges were developed and validated across several global populations; causes of controllable and uncontrollable preanalytical variation have been well described, and the clinical significance of bone turnovers in response to countless conditions has been studied.

C-TERMINAL TELOPEPTIDE OF TYPE I COLLAGEN

CTX is the carboxyterminal telopeptide of type I collagen that is cleaved off during osteoclast cathepsin-K–mediated bone resorption.[11] It measures bone resorption activity. It is relatively stable and decreases rapidly with antiresorptive therapy. It should be drawn fasting before 10 AM in the morning because it decreases postprandially, and it has diurnal variation with nadir from 11 AM to 3 PM in the afternoon.[10,12,13] It is falsely high with limited clinical utility in patients with severe renal impairment and may be 5 times higher in patients on hemodialysis.[14] CTX is less stable than PINP at room temperature and should be frozen as soon as possible. It may be measured in serum or plasma but is more stable in EDTA plasma especially when it is stored at room temperature for several hours before testing.[15]

N-TERMINAL PROPEPTIDE OF TYPE I COLLAGEN

PINP is the aminoterminal propeptide of type I collagen that is cleaved off when osteoblasts secrete type I collagen to form the osteoid framework of bones. It measures bone formation activity.[16] It is a stable assay with relatively good precision and low intraindividual variability.[10,17] When cleaved, PINP is a trimer, and it converts to a monomeric form. The trimer is hepatically cleared, and the monomeric form is renally cleared so PINP may be slightly increased in patients on hemodialysis in assays that measure the monomeric form along with the trimer.[18] PINP is superior to bone-specific alkaline phosphatase for monitoring osteoporosis therapy because trending PINP in response to osteoporosis therapy more consistently has an effect greater than the least significant change that would be expected with random variation.[19] PINP is falsely increased in patients with significant active hepatic, cardiac, or pulmonary fibrosis. It varies less with diurnal variation and food than CTX.[15]

OTHER BONE TURNOVER MARKERS

Other biochemical markers of bone formation include bone-specific alkaline phosphatase, C-terminal propeptide of type I collagen, and osteocalcin. Other biochemical markers of bone resorption include N-terminal telopeptide of type I collagen, pyridinolines, and tartrate-resistant acid phosphatase 5b (TRACP5b). These other bone turnover markers are summarized elsewhere and are currently less clinically relevant except for a couple of exceptions discussed later.[15,20]

Bone-specific alkaline phosphatase is useful as a marker of bone formation in certain specific scenarios. It is more widely available than PINP and is similarly a stable laboratory assay. It is not increased in response to impaired renal function, so it may have a role in patients with impaired renal function. It does not show significant changes in response to circadian rhythm or in response to food, similarly to PINP.[17] It can be used in situations when active fibrosis has falsely elevated PINP. However, if hepatic fibrosis has falsely elevated PINP, then bone-specific alkaline phosphatase may also be falsely elevated because there is 20% cross-reactivity with liver alkaline phosphatase.[15,17]

TRACP5b reflects the number of osteoclasts rather than osteoclast activity. It does not change with renal function, unlike CTX, so it may have a theoretic role for measurement of bone resorption in patients with impaired renal function. TRACP5b also appears to be more predictive of bony metastases in breast cancer than CTX.[21] However, TRACP5b is practically limited by its poor stability at room temperature and even while frozen. It is less stable in serum than plasma because platelets release TRACP during clotting.[15]

CAUSES OF PREANALYTIC VARIABILITY IN BONE TURNOVER MARKERS

CTX and other bone resorption markers[15] have a clinically significant circadian rhythm as noted above and should be drawn between 7:30 AM and 10 AM in the morning. PINP has minimal circadian rhythm variation and may be drawn all day during a clinic. Bone-specific alkaline phosphatase has more diurnal variation than PINP.[22] CTX decreases by about 50% postprandially.[12] PINP does not significantly decrease after meals. Bone resorption decreases during the luteal phase and increases in the late follicular phase of the menstrual cycle.[23] Bone turnover markers increase in winter as compared with summer, although there may be some contribution from changing vitamin D levels in temperate climates during different times of year.[24] The microbiome may affect bone turnover markers. Higher rates of *Klebsiella*, *Allisonella*, and *Megasphaera* in fecal bacteria correlate with higher PINP and CTX levels.[25] Intense exercise increases bone turnover formation and decreases bone turnover resorption.[26] Alcohol before blood draw acutely decreases bone turnover markers.[22] Degree of alcohol intake chronically over the past month progressively further decreases PINP but not CTX.[27] Impaired renal function causes most biochemical markers of resorption to increase. The preferred bone turnover markers for impaired renal function are PINP, bone-specific alkaline phosphatase, and TRACP5b. Higher bone turnover markers are seen in menopause. Age-adjusted reference intervals are important for interpretation of bone turnover markers. Bone turnover markers acutely decrease after a fracture for a few hours because of stress-related cortisol production, then increase for 4 months following fractures, and they decrease back to normal by 6 to 12 months following a fracture.[28-30]

MEDICAL CONDITIONS WITH LOW BONE TURNOVER

Growth hormone deficiency is a low bone turnover state, and severity of growth hormone deficiency is correlated with worsening bone density. The high prevalence of osteoporosis in patients with traumatic brain injuries may be related to the high prevalence of growth hormone deficiency.[31,32] Bone turnover is decreased in obesity, but this does not correlate with fractures. The effects of obesity on bone turnover markers are reversible with weight loss.[33,34] PINP and CTX are both decreased in type 2 diabetes.[35-39] The decrease in bone turnover markers in diabetes may be related to the decreased enzymatic cross-linking of type I collagen by lysyl oxidase that occurs in diabetes.[40,41] Decreased bone turnover is seen in both biochemical hypothyroidism and hypoparathyroidism.[15] Rapid decrease in bone turnover is seen after parathyroidectomy.[42]

MEDICAL CONDITIONS WITH HIGH BONE TURNOVER

Metastatic bone disease, which is common in breast cancer and prostate cancer, is associated with elevated bone turnover markers. Higher bone turnover marker levels are associated with higher rates of skeletal related events, disease progression, and death.[15,21] Heart failure, diastolic cardiomyopathy, and systemic sclerosis may falsely increase bone turnover markers by causing remodeling of the collagen matrix because both CTX and PINP are collagen based.[16] Primary hyperparathyroidism is associated with elevated bone turnover.[42] Vitamin D deficiency and calcium deficiency cause an increase of bone turnover markers, which can be a sign of osteomalacia. Bariatric surgery and other conditions that cause decreased absorption like chronic pancreatitis increase bone turnover.[22] Paget disease increases all bone turnover markers. Natural menopause and surgical menopause with bilateral oophorectomy increase bone turnover markers. Pregnancy increases bone turnover markers 2 to 3 times the normal range and are highest in the third trimester.[16] Immobility of any cause has been shown to increase bone turnover markers and has been seen in spinal cord patients, elderly patients, and critically ill patients.[43–45] Patients with acromegaly have elevated bone turnover markers and elevated fracture risk despite having normal to elevated bone density on DXA scans.[46,47] Treatment of acromegaly reduces and normalizes CTX but does not affect PINP levels. The increased risk of vertebral fracture does not normalize after treatment of acromegaly, suggesting durable impairment of bone quality.[46]

MEDICAL CONDITIONS WITH PREDOMINANTLY HIGH BONE RESORPTION

Anorexia nervosa increases bone resorption with low markers of bone formation when untreated. The effects on bone turnover are reversible with weight gain.[48] Multiple myeloma is associated with increased bone resorption and variable effects on bone formation.[49] CTX elevation has been shown to correlate with the presence and severity of bone lesions in multiple myeloma. Serial monitoring with CTX levels in multiple myeloma can also predict poor response to therapy when CTX is increasing or good response to therapy when CTX is decreasing.[50] Humoral hypercalcemia of malignancy increases markers of bone resorption and has variable effects on markers of bone formation. Rheumatoid arthritis is associated with an imbalance of bone resorption greater than bone formation.[15] Cushing is associated with elevated bone resorption and decreased or normal bone formation.[15] Mild autonomous cortisol secretion (MACS) is associated with a 4-fold increased risk of vertebral fractures compared with patients with nonfunctioning adrenal incidentalomas, but this increased risk is not predicted by DXA scan, suggesting excess cortisol impairs bone quality. MACS is not associated with a statistically different CTX or PINP than incidental nonfunctioning adrenal tumors, although patients with MACS do have significantly lower sclerostin levels, and degree of cortisol elevation is negatively correlated with sclerostin. Sclerostin normalizes and PINP increases after adrenalectomy in patients with MACS.[51] Acute liver disease is associated with increased bone resorption, and late fibrotic liver disease is also associated with falsely elevated PINP owing to increased hepatic synthesis and decreased hepatic clearance.[15]

MEDICATIONS AND BONE TURNOVER

Vitamin D and calcium supplementation decrease bone turnover. Exogenous corticosteroids decrease PINP and transiently increase bone resorption, but these effects are dependent on the dose of the corticosteroid. PINP is not useful for monitoring therapy in glucocorticoid-induced osteoporosis because it is decreased in response to steroids.[52] Estrogens decrease bone turnover markers, and progesterone increases bone formation markers. Aromatase inhibitors increase bone turnover markers by as much as 30%.[16] Androgen deprivation therapy increases bone turnover, and the effect can be reversed by bisphosphonates.[53] Thiazide diuretics transiently decrease bone turnover markers.[16] Pioglitazone decreases PINP.[15] Heparin decreases markers of bone formation. Warfarin decreases osteocalcin by increasing undercarboxylated osteocalcin but does not affect other bone turnover markers.[54] Biotin supplementation has been previously described to affect biotinylated thyroid stimulating hormone (TSH), parathyroid hormone, and troponin laboratory assays. Some bone turnover marker laboratory assays are biotinylated and are also at risk of being affected by biotin supplementation.[55,56] Large doses of biotin should be held for 72 hours before testing.

STATISTICAL INTERPRETATION OF BONE TURNOVER MARKERS

Bone turnover markers can vary from 1 measurement to the next both because of imprecision in laboratory assays and because of biological variation even when they are drawn correctly. Clinical significance for an individual patient requires knowledge of what change is statistically significant for the laboratory assay that is being used. Least significant change, also known as reference critical difference or reference change value, is a measure of what percentage change between 1 test to the next is greater than what would be expected with natural variation. Least significant change is calculated by multiplying 2.77, 1.96 × √2, times the coefficient of variation for the laboratory assay when it is equally likely for the bone turnover marker to increase or decrease versus 2.33, 1.65 × √2, times the coefficient of variation when the bone turnover marker is expected to go just in 1 direction like with bisphosphonate treatment, when bone turnover markers are expected to decrease.[57] The coefficient of variation for each individual laboratory assay can be provided by each laboratory or can be extrapolated from independent studies.

Independently determined coefficient of variation has been published for CTX laboratory assays at 4 large US commercial laboratories. In that 2019 analysis, the Labcorp electrochemiluminescence immunoassay (ECLIA) Immunodiagnostic Systems CTX laboratory performed worse than its competitors with a least significant change of 37% to 44%. The ARUP, Mayo, and Quest ECLIA Roche CTX laboratories had the least significant change less than 25% except for 1 outlier at Quest.[58] That means that change in CTX greater than 25% from 1 measurement to the next for most CTX laboratory assays is a statistically significant change and that change less than 25% should be considered statistically stable.

The TRIO study, initially published in 2011, determined the least significant change in their study as 29% for the IDS PINP laboratory, 23% for the Roche PINP laboratory, 54% for the IDS CTX laboratory, and 50% for the Roche CTX laboratory.[59,60] However, a 2020 paper reviewed the TRIO study data and concluded they overestimated the least significant change based on methodological flaws, including incorrectly using the 2.77 times coefficient of variation equation instead of the 2.33 times the coefficient of variation equation in a clinical situation where bone turnovers are expected to decrease on bisphosphonate therapy. Their revised least significant change for the TRIO study was 18% for PINP and 30% for CTX, although it is unclear if these values that were determined in a postmenopausal population in the TRIO study are externally valid to other populations.[57]

Trending of bone turnovers should be performed on the same laboratory assay. However, efforts are ongoing to harmonize the results for PINP across laboratory assays.[61]

FRACTURE RISK PREDICTION

Bone turnover markers do not have a role in diagnosis of osteoporosis on their own. Osteoporosis is diagnosed on DXA or by fracture history. In the TRIO study, only 20% of patients with osteoporosis diagnosed on DXA scan had a CTX above the upper limit of normal.[62] However, most fractures occur in people without osteoporosis, so clinical interest exists in finding patients at high risk for fractures without osteoporosis.

Bone turnover markers do have a role in fracture prediction, which has been consistent across multiple meta-analyses. The fracture prediction appears to be more effective over the short term in studies less than 7 years in duration than in the long term in studies greater than 10 years in duration.[15] When the IOF and the IFCC chose PINP and CTX as the preferred bone turnover markers in 2010, they reviewed the relationship between bone turnover markers and fracture and found that 18 out of 22 studies found at least 1 bone turnover marker associated with fracture risk.[10] These early studies were hampered by nonstandard outcomes, nonstandard bone turnover markers, and inability to limit controllable preanalytical variation, including fasting and diurnal variation.

The IOF and IFCC performed another meta-analysis in 2014 using the preferred bone turnover markers PINP and CTX and found a modest statistically significant association between elevated bone turnover markers and future fracture. They found each standard deviation increase in CTX was associated with a hazard ratio of 1.18 (95% confidence interval [CI]: 1.05–1.34) for fracture, and each standard deviation increase in PINP was associated with a hazard ratio of 1.23 (95% CI: 1.09–1.39).[63] This study's limitations included different laboratory assays used in the various individual trials and lack of adjustment for bone mineral density.

In a meta-analysis reviewing trials up to August 2018, increases in PINP and CTX per standard deviation were similarly predictive of fracture with a hazard ratio of 1.2 (95% CI: 1.05–1.37) for CTX and 1.28 (95% CI: 1.15–1.42) for PINP.[64] A weakness of this meta-analysis is they included older studies whereby bone turnovers were drawn in a nonfasting state.

Fracture prediction may be better using CTX and PINP together as opposed to separately as seen in a Singaporean population.[65] Despite modest fracture prediction, bone turnover markers have not been included in commonly used fracture risk algorithms like the FRAX or Garvan calculators.

FRACTURE PREDICTION IN HIGH-RISK POPULATIONS

One clinical population where we would benefit from more robust fracture prediction is in patients with diabetes because DXA underestimates fracture risk. Unfortunately, PINP and CTX were not predictive of fractures in patients with diabetes in the Health ABC study. That study did show similar fracture prediction ability for PINP and CTX in patients with prediabetes as compared with patients without diabetes or prediabetes. A 20% increase in PINP and CTX was associated with a 14% and 8% increase in fractures, respectively, in prediabetes, which was equivalent to the control group without diabetes.[35] Another clinical population at high risk for fracture is kidney-transplant recipients, who have a risk of fracture 4 times the general population. Baseline PINP before kidney transplant was found to be higher in patients who had a fracture, but this difference was not statistically or clinically significant so bone turnover markers cannot predict which kidney-transplant recipients are at high risk of future fracture.[66] Bone turnover markers also do not appear to be able to predict which patients on hemodialysis are at risk for high bone turnover or adynamic bone disease. In an Asian population, the 2 bone turnover markers that are not affected by renal function, bone specific alkaline phosphatase and TRACP5b, had a sensitivity to predict high bone turnover disease around 0.5, or no better than flipping a coin.[67]

MONITORING BISPHOSPHONATE THERAPY

The strongest clinical use of bone turnover markers is for monitoring response to antiresorptive therapies because less than half of patients prescribed a bisphosphonate are still taking it at 1 year, which is associated with poor outcomes and high costs.[7,68] Bone turnover markers are effective at monitoring the large bone turnover changes that occur with adherence to therapy. CTX suppresses by 50% to 80% within 2 months in patients started on bisphosphonate therapy, and PINP suppresses by approximately 40% to 60% within 6 months.[68,69] This response is well above least significant change as documented above for both bone turnover markers.

Several studies have shown bone turnover marker suppression on bisphosphonates predicts decreased fracture risk.[70] A meta-regression found short-term bone turnover marker treatment-related changes to be more predictive of vertebral fractures than nonvertebral fractures.[71] In a pooled analysis of several randomized control antiresorptive trials, short-term changes in bone turnover markers accounted for most of the treatment effect for preventing vertebral fractures but not for nonvertebral fractures.[72]

A guideline from the IOF and the European Calcified Tissue Society recommends checking PINP and CTX 3 months after initiation of antiresorptive therapy and evaluating for nonadherence, administration technique errors, or secondary causes of osteoporosis in patients whose bone turnover markers do not decrease more than least significant change.[68,73] For patients that do not have baseline bone turnover markers available before therapy, 1 strategy is to aim for bone turnover markers in the lower half of the normal reference range.[68] Another strategy is to aim for a CTX target less than 250 pg/mL based on extrapolation to CTX from a clinical urinary NTX fracture study. Based on expert opinion, the CTX target is less than 300 pg/mL, and the PINP target is less than 32 μg/L.[74] In an Australian prospective observational study, patients with bone turnover higher than these cutoffs were found to have an increased risk of fractures with an odds ratio (OR) of 1.7 to 2.1 for different subsets of their study population.[75]

ROLE IN BISPHOSPHONATE HOLIDAY

A clinical need exists to have objective data to guide the benefit and risks of bisphosphonate holidays. Suppression of bone turnover for too long can increase the rare side effect of an atypical femur fracture or osteonecrosis of the jaw (ONJ) but restarting a bisphosphonate holiday too soon or not stopping it early enough increases the risk of far more common typical femur fractures. The risk of fractures in bisphosphonate holidays is higher than in clinical trials.[76,77] Bone turnover markers, which increase long before a repeat DXA scan, guide clinical therapy to assess appropriateness of starting a bisphosphonate holiday and are widely used by clinicians. Widespread clinical use for guiding bisphosphonate holidays can be inferred from real-world US insurance claim data that show the decision to restart osteoporosis treatment within 30 days of bone turnover marker testing was associated with an OR of 2.67 (95% CI: 2.51–2.93).[9] The trial evidence supporting this clinical effort is sparse but has been slowly growing. A post hoc analysis of the FLEX extension of the FIT trial found CTX and bone-specific alkaline phosphatase had a hazard ratio of about 1.3 for predicting fracture during bisphosphonate holidays. The result was not statistically significant, but the study was underpowered to study this question. It also had external validity concerns because it underestimated the patients in the real world that have inadequate response to antiresorptive therapy before the start of a bisphosphonate holiday as seen in a retrospective analysis with a nonpreferred bone turnover marker and another with the preferred bone turnover marker, CTX.[78,79] More recently, the PROSA study has shown that a 30% increase in CTX 3 months after alendronate discontinuation predicts bone mineral density decrease at 1 year after alendronate discontinuation.[80]

Bone turnover markers may have a role in predicting patients at risk of ONJ. In a population of 950 patients on bisphosphonate therapy undergoing dental extractions, only 4 patients had ONJ, and all 4 patients had a CTX less than 150 pg/mL. This barely missed statistical significance with a *P* value of .073 but was likely underpowered because of the rarity of ONJ. Even in patients with CTX less than 150 pg/mL, the risk of ONJ was only 2%.[81]

MONITORING DENOSUMAB THERAPY

CTX drops to near undetectable levels within days on denosumab treatment, and PINP reaches a nadir in 3 to 6 months, so monitoring adherence is very easy with bone turnover markers if clinically required.[82] Bone turnover markers rapidly increase by 9 months after the last denosumab injection and can remain elevated for up to 30 months, which can be associated with rebound compression fractures.[83] Prevention of these rebound fractures is where bone turnover markers are clinically useful in denosumab therapy because the timing for when bone turnovers start increasing is variable after the end of denosumab therapy. Transition to bisphosphonate therapy too early before bone turnovers start to increase or too late after rapid increase can result in rebound fractures. The Endocrine Society recommends using bone turnover markers to guide transitions off of denosumab therapy, although further evidence is needed.[83]

MONITORING ANABOLIC THERAPY

PINP quickly increases in response to teriparatide and abaloparatide and peaks after 3 months. CTX does not peak until several months later. Per expert opinion, PINP increasing by greater than 10 µg/L above baseline is reassuring for therapy adherence and efficacy of treatment.[68] Romosozumab increases PINP and decreases CTX. The role of bone turnover markers in transitions from antiresorptive therapy to anabolic therapy appears limited. In patients transitioning from bisphosphonate therapy to anabolic teriparatide or romosozumab, increase in PINP greater than 10 µg/L did not predict changes in bone mineral density.[84]

SUMMARY

The clinical use of bone turnover markers is growing because they help fill clinical gaps in osteoporosis management. The designation of preferred bone turnover markers, the development of reference intervals, and the development of therapeutic targets have improved their clinical utility. When used effectively with understanding of their limitations, they can expedite clinical response to therapeutic decisions, assess adherence to medical therapies, suggest secondary causes of osteoporosis, and modulate fracture risk prediction. Bone turnover marker testing has even been shown to be associated with lower risk of fracture compared with patients who were not tested (OR, 0.87; 95% CI: 0.85–0.88) in US insurance claim data.[9] Areas of future research that can further improve the clinical applicability of bone turnover markers include studying fracture data in bisphosphonate holidays directed by bone turnover monitoring and prospective trials that validate current expert opinion-based therapeutic targets for bone turnover markers.

CLINICS CARE POINTS

Guide to Ordering Bone Turnover Markers
- Use preferred bone turnover markers, PINP and CTX, for most situations.

- Draw laboratory tests fasting in the morning from 7:30 AM to 10:00 AM (required for CTX but not for PINP).
- Advise alcohol avoidance the day before the blood draw and avoid excessive alcohol in the month before the blood draw.
- Advise excessive exercise avoidance the day before the blood draw.
- Hold biotin supplements for 72 hours before the blood draw.
- Draw laboratory tests in the follicular phase of the menstrual cycle in the first week after last menstrual period for premenopausal women.
- Trend the same laboratory assay drawn at the same facility from the same laboratory company.
- Compare laboratory tests drawn at the same time of year in temperate regions.
- Freeze CTX as soon as possible after laboratory draw.
- Draw CTX in EDTA plasma if the laboratory draw will be at room temperature for more than a few hours if EDTA plasma is accepted at your laboratory facility.
- Improve diabetes control to improve accuracy of bone turnover markers.
- Avoid CTX with poor renal function.

Interpreting and Adjusting Therapy with Bone Turnover Markers

- Changes in bone turnover markers greater than about 20% for PINP and about 25% to 30% for CTX are significant and greater than least significant change.
- Consider asking your laboratory for the coefficient of variation for your laboratory assay and use formula 2.33 × coefficient of variation to calculate your laboratory assay's least significant change percentage.
- If pretreatment bone turnover markers are not available, aim to reduce bone turnover markers to the lower half of the normal reference range or less than 250 to 300 pg/mL for CTX and less than 32 μg/L for PINP on antiresorptive therapy.
- When bone turnover markers do not suppress, investigate for poor adherence, inappropriate medication administration, low dietary calcium or vitamin D, other secondary causes of osteoporosis, occult fractures in the past 6 months, and confounding conditions that affect type I collagen metabolism like severe liver fibrosis.
- Check bone turnover markers 3 to 6 months after therapeutic interventions to assess for efficacy.

DISCLOSURE

The author has nothing to disclose.

REFERENCES

1. Epidemiology. International Osteoporosis Foundation website. Available at: https://www.osteoporosis.foundation/health-professionals/fragility-fractures/epidemiology. Accessed February 3, 2021.
2. Burge R, Dawson-Hughes B, Solomon D, et al. Incidence and economic burden of osteoporosis-related fractures in the United States, 2005-2025. J Bone Miner Res 2006;22(3):465–75.
3. Wu C, Chang Y, Chen C, et al. Consensus statement on the use of bone turnover markers for short-term monitoring of osteoporosis treatment in the Asia-Pacific region. J Clin Densitom 2021;24(1):3–13.

4. Siris E, Chen Y, Abbott T, et al. Bone mineral density thresholds for pharmacological intervention to prevent fractures. Arch Intern Med 2004;164(10):1108.
5. Balasubramanian A, Zhang J, Chen L, et al. Risk of subsequent fracture after prior fracture among older women. Osteoporos Int 2018;30(1):79–92.
6. Fitzpatrick L. Secondary causes of osteoporosis. Mayo Clin Proc 2002;77(5): 453–68.
7. Warriner A, Curtis J. Adherence to osteoporosis treatments: room for improvement. Curr Opin Rheumatol 2009;21(4):356–62.
8. Sharman Moser S, Yu J, Goldshtein I, et al. Cost and consequences of nonadherence with oral bisphosphonate therapy. Ann Pharmacother 2016;50(4):262–9.
9. Lane NE, Saag K, O'Neill TJ, et al. Real-world bone turnover marker use: impact on treatment decisions and fracture. Osteoporos Int 2020. https://doi.org/10.1007/s00198-020-05734-0.
10. Vasikaran S, Cooper C, Eastell R, et al. International Osteoporosis Foundation and International Federation of Clinical Chemistry and Laboratory Medicine position on bone marker standards in osteoporosis. Clin Chem Lab Med 2011;49(8): 1271–4.
11. Garnero P, Ferreras M, Karsdal M, et al. The type I collagen fragments ICTP and CTX reveal distinct enzymatic pathways of bone collagen degradation. J Bone Miner Res 2003;18(5):859–67.
12. Clowes JA, Hannon RA, Yap TS, et al. Effect of feeding on bone turnover markers and its impact on biological variability of measurements. Bone 2002;30(6): 886–90.
13. Wichers M, Schmidt E, Bidlingmaier F, et al. Diurnal rhythm of CrossLaps in human serum. Clin Chem 1999;45(10):1858–60.
14. Delanaye P, Souberbielle J, Lafage-Proust M, et al. Can we use circulating biomarkers to monitor bone turnover in CKD haemodialysis patients? Hypotheses and facts. Nephrol Dial Transplant 2014;29(5):997–1004.
15. Szulc P. Bone turnover: biology and assessment tools. Best Pract Res Clin Endocrinol Metab 2018;32(5):725–38.
16. Greenblatt MB, Tsai JN, Wein MN. Bone turnover markers in the diagnosis and monitoring of metabolic bone disease. Clin Chem 2017;63(2):464–74.
17. Wheater G, Elshahaly M, Tuck SP, et al. The clinical utility of bone marker measurements in osteoporosis. J Transl Med 2013;11(1):201.
18. Koivula M, Ruotsalainen V, Björkman M, et al. Difference between total and intact assays for N-terminal propeptide of type I procollagen reflects degradation of pN-collagen rather than denaturation of intact propeptide. Ann Clin Biochem 2010;47(1):67–71.
19. Brown JP, Albert C, Nassar BA, et al. Bone turnover markers in the management of postmenopausal osteoporosis. Clin Biochem 2009;42(10):929–42.
20. Jain S, Camacho P. Use of bone turnover markers in the management of osteoporosis. Curr Opin Endocrinol Diabetes Obes 2018;25(6):366–72.
21. Lumachi F, Basso SMM, Camozzi V, et al. Clinica chimica acta. Clin Chim Acta 1956;460:227–30.
22. Eastell R, Szulc P. Use of bone turnover markers in postmenopausal osteoporosis. Lancet Diabetes Endocrinol 2017;5(11):908–23.
23. Gorai I, Chaki O, Nakayama M, et al. Urinary biochemical markers for bone resorption during the menstrual cycle. Calcif Tissue Int 1995;57(2):100–4.
24. Thiering E, Brüske I, Kratzsch J, et al. Associations between serum 25-hydroxyvitamin D and bone turnover markers in a population based sample of German children. Sci Rep 2015;5(1):18138.

25. He J, Xu S, Zhang B, et al. Gut microbiota and metabolite alterations associated with reduced bone mineral density or bone metabolic indexes in postmenopausal osteoporosis. Aging 2020;12(9):8583–604.

26. Gombos Császár G, Bajsz V, Sió E, et al. The direct effect of specific training and walking on bone metabolic markers in young adults with peak bone mass. Acta Physiol Hung 2014;101(2):205–15.

27. Kim TW, Ventura AS, Winter MR, et al. Alcohol and bone turnover markers among people living with HIV and substance use disorder. Alcohol Clin Exp Res 2020; 44(4):992–1000.

28. Stoffel K, Engler H, Kuster M, et al. Changes in biochemical markers after lower limb fractures. Clin Chem 2007;53(1):131–4.

29. Ivaska KK, Gerdhem P, Åkesson K, et al. Effect of fracture on bone turnover markers: a longitudinal study comparing marker levels before and after injury in 113 elderly women. J Bone Miner Res 2007;22(8):1155–64.

30. Højsager FD, Rand MS, Pedersen SB, et al. Fracture-induced changes in bio-markers CTX, PINP, OC, and BAP—a systematic review. Osteoporos Int 2019; 30(12):2381–9.

31. Bajwa NM, Kesavan C, Mohan S. Long-term consequences of traumatic brain injury in bone metabolism. Front Neurol 2018;9:115.

32. Colao A, Di Somma C, Pivonello R, et al. Bone loss is correlated to the severity of growth hormone deficiency in adult patients with hypopituitarism. J Clin Endocrinol Metab 1999;84(6):1919–24.

33. Cohen A, Dempster DW, Recker RR, et al. Abdominal fat is associated with lower bone formation and inferior bone quality in healthy premenopausal women: a transiliac bone biopsy study. J Clin Endocrinol Metab 2013;98(6):2562–72.

34. Evans AL, Paggiosi MA, Eastell R, et al. Bone density, microstructure and strength in obese and normal weight men and women in younger and older adulthood. J Bone Miner Res 2015;30(5):920–8.

35. Napoli N, Conte C, Eastell R, et al. Bone turnover markers do not predict fracture risk in type 2 diabetes. J Bone Miner Res 2020;35(12):2363–71.

36. Shu A, Shu A, Yin M, et al. Bone structure and turnover in type 2 diabetes mellitus. Osteoporos Int 2012;23(2):635–41.

37. Dobnig H, Piswanger-Solkner JC, Roth M, et al. Type 2 diabetes mellitus in nursing home patients: effects on bone turnover, bone mass, and fracture risk. J Clin Endocrinol Metab 2006;91(9):3355–63.

38. Gerdhem P, Isaksson A, Åkesson K, et al. Increased bone density and decreased bone turnover, but no evident alteration of fracture susceptibility in elderly women with diabetes mellitus. Osteoporos Int 2005;16(12):1506–12.

39. Krakauer JC, Mckenna MJ, Buderer NF, et al. Bone loss and bone turnover in diabetes. Diabetes 1995;44(7):775–82.

40. Saito M, Fujii K, Mori Y, et al. Role of collagen enzymatic and glycation induced cross-links as a determinant of bone quality in spontaneously diabetic WBN/Kob rats. Osteoporos Int 2006;17(10):1514–23.

41. Khosravi R, Sodek KL, Faibish M, et al. Collagen advanced glycation inhibits its discoidin domain receptor 2 (DDR2)-mediated induction of lysyl oxidase in osteoblasts. Bone 2013;58:33–41.

42. Rajeev P, Movseysan A, Baharani A. Changes in bone turnover markers in primary hyperparathyroidism and response to surgery. Ann R Coll Surg Engl 2017;99(7):559–62.

43. Orford N, Cattigan C, Brennan S, et al. The association between critical illness and changes in bone turnover in adults: a systematic review. Osteoporos Int 2014;25(10):2335–46.
44. Gifre L, Vidal J, Carrasco J, et al. Risk factors for the development of osteoporosis after spinal cord injury. A 12-month follow-up study. Osteoporos Int 2015;26(9): 2273–80.
45. Chen JS, Cameron ID, Cumming RG, et al. Effect of age-related chronic immobility on markers of bone turnover. J Bone Miner Res 2006;21(2):324–31.
46. Constantin T, Tangpricha V, Shah R, et al. Calcium and bone turnover markers in acromegaly: a prospective, controlled study. J Clin Endocrinol Metab 2017; 102(7):2416–24.
47. Mazziotti G, Biagioli E, Maffezzoni F, et al. Bone turnover, bone mineral density, and fracture risk in acromegaly: a meta-analysis. J Clin Endocrinol Metab 2015;100(2):384–94.
48. Fazeli PK, Klibanski A. Anorexia nervosa and bone metabolism. Bone 2014;66: 39–45.
49. Terpos E, Dimopoulos MA, Palumbo A, et al. The use of biochemical markers of bone remodeling in multiple myeloma: a report of the International Myeloma Working Group. Leukemia 2010;24(10):1700–12.
50. Auzina D, Erts R, Lejniece S. Prognostic value of the bone turnover markers in multiple myeloma. Exp Oncol 2017;39(1):53–6.
51. Athimulam S, Delivanis D, Thomas M, et al. The impact of mild autonomous cortisol secretion on bone turnover markers. J Clin Endocrinol Metab 2020; 105(5):1469–77.
52. Chotiyarnwong P, McCloskey EV. Pathogenesis of glucocorticoid-induced osteoporosis and options for treatment. Nat Rev Endocrinol 2020;16(8):437–47.
53. Wang A, Karunasinghe N, Lindsay P, et al. Effect of androgen deprivation therapy on bone mineral density in a prostate cancer cohort in New Zealand: a pilot study. *Clinical Medicine Insights*. Oncology 2017;11. 1179554917733449.
54. Knapen MHJ, Hellemons-Boode BSP, Langenberg-Ledeboer M, et al. Effect of oral anticoagulant treatment on markers for calcium and bone metabolism. Pathophysiol Haemost Thromb 2001;30(6):290–7.
55. Marcius M, Vrkić N, Getaldić-Švarc B. Analytical evaluation of P1NP assay, a biochemical marker of bone turnover. Biochem Med 2006;16(2):178–90.
56. Biotin: interference with laboratory assays. Quest Diagnostics Education Center Web site. Available at: https://education.questdiagnostics.com/faq/FAQ202. Accessed Feb 15, 2021.
57. Tan RZ, Loh TP, Vasikaran S. Bone turnover marker monitoring in osteoporosis treatment response. Eur J Endocrinol 2020;183(1):C5–7.
58. Hindi SM, Vittinghoff E, Schafer AL, et al. Commercial laboratory reproducibility of serum CTX in clinical practice. JBMR Plus 2019;3(10):e10225.
59. Netelenbos JC, Geusens PP, Ypma G, et al. Adherence and profile of non-persistence in patients treated for osteoporosis-a large-scale, long-term retrospective study in the Netherlands. Osteoporos Int 2011;22(5):1537–46.
60. Eastell R, Pigott T, Gossiel F, et al. Diagnosis of endocrine disease: bone turnover markers: are they clinically useful? Eur J Endocrinol 2018;178(1):R19–31.
61. Vasikaran SD, Bhattoa HP, Eastell R, et al. Harmonization of commercial assays for PINP; the way forward. Osteoporos Int 2020;31(3):409–12.
62. Naylor K, Naylor K, Jacques R, et al. Response of bone turnover markers to three oral bisphosphonate therapies in postmenopausal osteoporosis: the TRIO study. Osteoporos Int 2016;27(1):21–31.

63. Johansson H, Odén A, Kanis J, et al. A meta-analysis of reference markers of bone turnover for prediction of fracture. Calcif Tissue Int 2014;94(5):560–7.

64. Tian A, Ma J, Feng K, et al. Reference markers of bone turnover for prediction of fracture: a meta-analysis. J Orthop Surg Res 2019;14(1):68.

65. Dai Z, Wang R, Ang L, et al. Bone turnover biomarkers and risk of osteoporotic hip fracture in an Asian population. Bone 2015;83:171–7.

66. Evenepoel P, Claes K, Meijers B, et al. Bone mineral density, bone turnover markers, and incident fractures in de novo kidney transplant recipients. Kidney Int 2019;95(6):1461–70.

67. Laowalert S, Khotavivattana T, Wattanachanya L, et al. Bone turnover markers predict type of bone histomorphometry and bone mineral density in Asian chronic haemodialysis patients. Nephrology 2020;25(2):163–71.

68. Lorentzon M, Branco J, Brandi M, et al. Algorithm for the use of biochemical markers of bone turnover in the diagnosis, assessment and follow-up of treatment for osteoporosis. Adv Ther 2019;36(10):2811–24.

69. Rosen CJ, Hochberg MC, Bonnick SL, et al. Treatment with once-weekly alendronate 70 mg compared with once-weekly risedronate 35 mg in women with postmenopausal osteoporosis: a randomized double-blind study. J Bone Miner Res 2005;20(1):141–51.

70. Vasikaran S, Vasikaran S, Eastell R, et al. Markers of bone turnover for the prediction of fracture risk and monitoring of osteoporosis treatment: a need for international reference standards. Osteoporos Int 2011;22(2):391–420.

71. Bauer DC, Black DM, Bouxsein ML, et al. Treatment-related changes in bone turnover and fracture risk reduction in clinical trials of anti-resorptive drugs: a meta-regression. J Bone Miner Res 2018;33(4):634–42.

72. Eastell R, Black DM, Lui L, et al. Treatment-related changes in bone turnover and fracture risk reduction in clinical trials of antiresorptive drugs: proportion of treatment effect explained. J Bone Miner Res 2020;36(2):236–43.

73. Diez-Perez A, Naylor KE, Abrahamsen B, et al, International Osteoporosis Foundation and European Calcified Tissue Society Working Group. Recommendations for the screening of adherence to oral bisphosphonates. Osteoporos Int 2017;28(3):767–74.

74. Chubb SAP, Byrnes E, Manning L, et al. Bone turnover markers: defining a therapeutic target. Clin Biochem 2017;50(3):162–3.

75. Fisher A, Fisher L, Srikusalanukul W, et al. Bone turnover status: classification model and clinical implications. Int J Med Sci 2018;15(4):323–38.

76. Chiha M, Myers LE, Ball CA, et al. Long-term follow-up of patients on drug holiday from bisphosphonates: real-world setting. Endocr Pract 2013;19(6):989–94.

77. Xu LHR, Adams-Huet B, Poindexter JR, et al. Determinants of change in bone mineral density and fracture risk during bisphosphonate holiday. Osteoporos Int 2016;27(5):1701–8.

78. Liel Y, Plakht Y, Tailakh MA. Bone turnover in osteoporotic women during longterm oral bisphosphonates treatment: implications for treatment failure and "drug holiday" in the real world. Endocr Pract 2017;23(7):787–93.

79. Statham L, Abdy S, Aspray TJ. Can bone turnover markers help to define the suitability and duration of bisphosphonate drug holidays? Drugs in context 2020;9:1–5.

80. Sølling AS, Harsløf T, Bruun NH, et al. The predictive value of bone turnover markers during discontinuation of alendronate: The PROSA study. Osteoporos Int 2021. https://doi.org/10.1007/s00198-021-05835-4. Available at: https://www.ncbi.nlm.nih.gov/pubmed/33517477.

81. Hutcheson A, Cheng A, Kunchar R, et al. A C-terminal crosslinking telopeptide test–based protocol for patients on oral bisphosphonates requiring extraction: a prospective single-center controlled study. J Oral Maxillofac Surg 2014;72(8): 1456–62.

82. Eastell R, Christiansen C, Grauer A, et al. Effects of denosumab on bone turnover markers in postmenopausal osteoporosis. J Bone Miner Res 2011;26(3):530–7.

83. Tsourdi E, Zillikens M, Meier C, et al. Fracture risk and management of discontinuation of denosumab therapy: a systematic review and position statement by ECTS. J Clin Endocrinol Metab 2020. https://doi.org/10.1210/clinem/dgaa756.

84. Takada J, Dinavahi R, Miyauchi A, et al. Relationship between P1NP, a biochemical marker of bone turnover, and bone mineral density in patients transitioned from alendronate to romosozumab or teriparatide: a post hoc analysis of the STRUCTURE trial. J Bone Miner Metab 2020;38(3):310–5.

Updates on Osteoporosis in Men

Dima L. Diab, MD, CCD[a],*, Nelson B. Watts, MD, MACE, CCD[b]

KEYWORDS

- Osteoporosis • Men • Fractures • Updates • Diagnosis • Evaluation • Treatment

KEY POINTS

- The incidence of osteoporosis in men increases with age, and, although typically thought of as a disease impacting women, the mortality associated with major fragility fractures is higher in men than women.
- As in women, the diagnosis of osteoporosis is established by measurement of bone mineral density by dual-energy x-ray absorptiometry of the spine, hip, and/or forearm (T-score of −2.5 or lower), or by the presence of a low-trauma or fragility fracture.
- Prior fracture and T-score −2.5 or below will identify only a small proportion of men at high risk of fracture; for men with T-scores between −1.0 and −2.5, a fracture risk assessment with FRAX or similar tool is essential.
- Contributing factors can be identified in up to 60% of men who have osteoporosis, and it is important to identify and address these factors to manage patients appropriately and prevent further bone loss.
- Several Food and Drug Administration–approved pharmacologic treatments shown to reduce fracture risk in women are also approved for men but, except for zoledronic acid, the studies in men were small, short, and had bone mineral density as opposed to fracture endpoints.

INTRODUCTION

Osteoporosis is defined as a generalized skeletal disorder characterized by compromised bone strength predisposing to an increased risk of fractures. Bone strength denotes the integration of 2 main features: bone density and bone quality.[1] Based on the Surgeon General's report on bone health and osteoporosis published in 2004, in the United States, osteoporosis affected 8 million women and 2 million men, with the

[a] Division of Endocrinology/Metabolism, Department of Internal Medicine, Cincinnati VA Medical Center, University of Cincinnati Bone Health and Osteoporosis, 231 Albert Sabin Way, MSB 7th Floor, Cincinnati, OH 45267, USA; [b] Mercy Health Osteoporosis and Bone Health Services, 4760 E. Galbraith Road, Suite 212, Cincinnati, OH 45236, USA
* Corresponding author.
E-mail address: diabd@ucmail.uc.edu

Endocrinol Metab Clin N Am 50 (2021) 239–249
https://doi.org/10.1016/j.ecl.2021.03.001
0889-8529/21/© 2021 Elsevier Inc. All rights reserved.

annual incidence of osteoporotic fractures exceeding 2 million and expected to rise to more than 3 million by the year 2020.[2]

EPIDEMIOLOGY

Osteoporosis is predominantly a condition of elderly individuals.[3] Both men and women lose bone mass with advancing age,[4] and the prevalence of osteoporosis increases in older adults.[5] It is currently estimated that approximately 5% of men in the United States have osteoporosis by T-score definition.[6] Although this is less common than in women, increasing attention is being paid to osteoporosis in men given the significant morbidity and mortality associated with this condition. As many as 1 in 4 men older than 50 years will develop at least 1 osteoporosis-related fracture in their lifetime.[7] Because men have greater bone mass than women, they typically present with an osteoporotic fracture approximately 10 years later than women.[8] In part because fractures in men occur at an older age than in women, mortality associated with hip fractures as well as other major fractures is higher in men than in women.[9] Even so, men are less likely than women to be evaluated or treated for osteoporosis after sustaining a fracture.[10]

DIAGNOSIS

As in women, the diagnosis of osteoporosis in men can be established by measurement of bone mineral density (BMD) by dual-energy x-ray absorptiometry of the spine, hip, and/or forearm (T-score of -2.5 or lower), although a clinical diagnosis can be made in individuals who sustain a low-trauma or fragility fracture (**Table 1**). The National Osteoporosis Foundation recommends BMD testing for all men 70 years and older. Testing should be done sooner (starting age 50) in men with risk factors for fracture such as hypogonadism, hypercalciuria, nutritional deficiencies, history of prior fracture, family history of osteoporosis, smoking, excessive alcohol intake, or long-term use of high-risk medications, for example, glucocorticoid therapy, anti-epilepsy drug therapy, or androgen deprivation therapy for prostate cancer.[11] The International Society for Clinical Densitometry recommends that BMD measurements alone should not be used to diagnose osteoporosis in men younger than 50 years, but emphasizes the need for a fracture risk assessment tool to identify men at high risk of fracture who do not yet meet the T-score criteria.[12]

EVALUATION

Potential contributing factors are found in up to 60% of men with osteoporosis.[13–15] Furthermore, these are found in 20% to 50% of patients with bone loss on

Table 1	
World Health Organization diagnostic classification of osteoporosis	
Category	**T-Score[a]**
Normal	-1.0 and above
Low bone mass (osteopenia)	Between -1.0 and -2.5
Osteoporosis	-2.5 and below

[a] The T-score compares an individual's bone mineral density with the mean value for young healthy individuals and expresses the difference as a standard deviation score.

From Diab DL, Watts NB. Diagnosis and treatment of osteoporosis in older adults. *Endocrinol Metab Clin North Am* 2013;42(2):305-317; with permission.

pharmacologic therapy.[16] The major factors are listed in **Table 2**. The evaluation of any patient with osteoporosis should begin with a history and physical examination including a review of the complete list of medications, because many of the contributing factors can be identified or excluded with a careful history and physical examination. Height (using a stadiometer) and weight should also be measured.

Initial laboratory testing should include the following:

- Complete blood count
- Complete metabolic panel including creatinine, calcium, phosphorus, alkaline phosphatase, and liver function tests
- 25-OH D to evaluate for vitamin D deficiency
- Testosterone (total and free) to test for hypogonadism
- Thyroid-stimulating hormone in symptomatic patients or in subjects on treatment for thyroid disease
- 24-hour urine calcium, sodium, and creatinine to check for calcium malabsorption or hypercalciuria

This workup identifies approximately 90% of occult disorders at a reasonable cost.[17] Several contributing factors, such as mild hyperparathyroidism or celiac disease, may be subtle; therefore, the presence of laboratory abnormalities on this initial workup may suggest certain etiologies and guide further diagnostic investigation.

TREATMENT
Nonpharmacologic Management

Lifestyle factors that contribute to bone loss, including smoking, excessive alcohol, physical inactivity, and poor nutrition, should be addressed. Measures aimed at fall prevention also should be encouraged. In addition, recommendations for adequate calcium and vitamin D supplementation should be discussed. Calcium intake should be approximately 1000 to 1200 mg per day.[18] The recommended total calcium intake for men age 70 and older is 1200 mg daily, with the preferred source being dietary[19,20]; supplementation is recommended if this cannot be obtained through diet alone. Low vitamin D is common, and supplementation may be important for the maintenance of bone and muscle strength.[21–23] Risk factors for vitamin D deficiency include low exposure to sunlight, among others,[24] and vitamin D replacement therapy has been shown to reduce body sway and decrease fall risk in older individuals,[25–28] as well as decrease fracture risk in men and women aged 65 years and older living in the community.[29] Vitamin D status is assessed by measurement of its major circulating metabolite, 25-hydroxy vitamin D.[30] It is recommend to maintain a serum 25-hydroxy vitamin D level of at least 30 ng/mL in men with osteoporosis.[31–33] Many patients require supplements of vitamin D, 2000 IU daily or more, to achieve this level.

Pharmacologic Management

Based on current guidelines,[11,18] health care providers should consider treating patients based on the following:

- T-score $\leq$−2.5 at the lumbar spine, femoral neck, total hip, or one-third distal radius (after appropriate evaluation to exclude secondary causes)
- A hip or vertebral (clinical or morphometric) fracture
- Low bone mass (T-score between −1.0 and −2.5) AND a 10-year probability of a hip fracture $\geq$3% OR a 10-year probability of a major osteoporosis-related fracture $\geq$20% using the FRAX Web-based tool (**Table 3**)

Table 2
Major causes of secondary osteoporosis

Endocrine/Metabolic Diseases	Nutritional Conditions	Drugs	Genetic Disorders	Miscellaneous
Hypogonadism	Vitamin D deficiency	Glucocorticoids	Osteogenesis imperfecta	Rheumatoid arthritis
Hypercalciuria	Calcium deficiency	Anti-epilepsy drugs	Homocystinuria	Inflammatory bowel disease
Hyperthyroidism	Vitamin B12 deficiency	Excess thyroid hormone	Ehlers-Danlos syndrome	COPD
Hyperparathyroidism	Weight loss	Androgen deprivation therapy	Marfan syndrome	Organ transplantation
Cushing syndrome	Malabsorption	Heparin	Glycogen storage diseases	Immobilization
Diabetes mellitus	Gastric surgery	Thiazolidinediones	Gaucher disease	Muscular dystrophy
	Chronic liver disease	Selective serotonin reuptake inhibitors	Hypophosphatasia	Multiple sclerosis
	Alcoholism	Proton pump inhibitors	Porphyria	Multiple myeloma
	Malnutrition	Excess vitamin A	Hemochromatosis	Some cancers (leukemia and lymphomas)
	Prolonged TPN	Cyclosporine		ESRD
				Mastocytosis
				Thalassemia
				Sickle cell disease
				HIV

Abbreviations: COPD, chronic obstructive pulmonary disease; ESRD, end-stage renal disease; HIV, human immunodeficiency virus; TPN, total parenteral nutrition.

Adapted from Camacho PM, Petak SM, Binkley N, et al. American Association of Clinical Endocrinologists/American College of Endocrinology Clinical Practice Guidelines for the Diagnosis and Treatment of Postmenopausal Osteoporosis – 2020 Update. *Endocr Pract.* 2020;26(Suppl 1):1-46; with permission.

Table 3
Clinical risk factors for fracture included in the Fracture Risk Assessment model (FRAX)

Current Age	Current Smoking
Gender	Alcohol intake (3 or more drinks/d)
Low body mass index (kg/m²)	Rheumatoid arthritis
A prior osteoporotic fracture (including morphometric vertebral fracture)	Secondary osteoporosis
Parental history of hip fracture	Femoral neck BMD
Oral glucocorticoids ≥5 mg/d of prednisone for ≥3 mo (ever)	

Abbreviation: BMD, bone mineral density.

From Diab DL, Watts NB. Diagnosis and treatment of osteoporosis in older adults. *Endocrinol Metab Clin North Am* 2013;42(2):305-317; with permission.

- Clinician's judgment and/or patient preferences may indicate treatment for people with 10-year fracture probabilities below these levels

Most men at high risk will be identified only by using a fracture risk assessment tool, such as FRAX.[34] The current Food and Drug Administration (FDA)-approved bone-active agents for osteoporosis in men and their available dosing forms are shown in **Table 4**.

Initial approval of pharmacologic agents for treatment of osteoporosis is usually based on studies of postmenopausal women with osteoporosis. Typically, these are 3-year placebo-controlled trials with new vertebral fracture as the primary endpoint. Important secondary endpoints are hip fractures and nonvertebral fractures. For approval in populations other than postmenopausal women with osteoporosis (such as men, or glucocorticoid-induced osteoporosis), so-called bridging studies are sufficient. These are too small and too short to show fracture reduction, but demonstration of similar gains in BMD in men compared with postmenopausal women are needed.

Bisphosphonates

Bisphosphonates reduce osteoclastic bone resorption by entering the osteoclast and causing loss of resorptive function as well as accelerating osteoclast apoptosis. Alendronate was the first bisphosphonate approved by the FDA for the treatment of

Table 4
Available dosing forms of Food and Drug Administration–approved bone-active agents for men with osteoporosis

	Oral			Intravenous Infusion	Subcutaneous Injection
Drug	Daily	Weekly	Monthly		
Alendronate (Fosamax)	5 and 10 mg	35 and 70 mg			
Risedronate (Actonel)	5 mg	35 mg	150 mg		
Zoledronic acid (Reclast)				5 mg per year	
Denosumab (Prolia)					60 mg q6 months
Teriparatide (Forteo)					20 μg daily

osteoporosis. A randomized double-blind trial in 241 men showed that alendronate increased spine and femoral neck BMD and with a suggestion that the incidence of vertebral fractures was reduced at 2 years.[35] Subsequent meta-analyses revealed similar findings.[36,37] Alendronate was also found to increase lumbar spine and hip BMD in men with glucocorticoid-induced osteoporosis,[38] as well as in those on androgen deprivation therapy.[39]

Similarly, an open-label 12-month study of risedronate showed an increase in spine and hip BMD and a reduction in vertebral fractures in men with osteoporosis.[40] An extension of this study showed that risedronate reduced vertebral and nonvertebral fractures in men with osteoporosis and that the effect was sustained over 2 years.[41] A randomized clinical trial of 284 men with osteoporosis comparing weekly risedronate with placebo also showed that risedronate increased lumbar spine BMD.[42]

Zoledronic acid is the only intravenous bisphosphonate that has demonstrated efficacy for fracture prevention in men in a placebo-controlled trial. In a multicenter, double-blind, trial of 1199 men with osteoporosis receiving annual intravenous zoledronic acid infusion or placebo over a period of 24 months, zoledronic acid treatment was associated with a significantly reduced risk of vertebral fracture.[43]

In a recent meta-analysis of several trials in men with osteoporosis, bisphosphonates reduced the risk of vertebral (relative risk [RR] 0.37, 95% confidence interval [CI] 0.25–0.54) and nonvertebral (RR 0.60, 95% CI 0.40–0.90) fractures.[44] However, more studies to confirm the antifracture efficacy of bisphosphonates in men with osteoporosis would be desirable, particularly regarding nonvertebral and hip fractures. Most studies had few such fractures and thus were underpowered to assess the effects on these clinical endpoints.[45] More data are also required regarding the potential long-term risks of antiresorptive therapy, including osteonecrosis of the jaw and atypical femur fractures (AFF). Although there is no robust evidence that the side-effect profile is different between men and women,[46] a Swedish study suggested that the risk of AFF is lower in men than in women.[47]

Denosumab

Denosumab is a fully human monoclonal antibody to the receptor activator of nuclear factor kappa-B ligand, an osteoclast differentiating factor. It inhibits osteoclast formation, thus decreasing bone resorption. Similar to bisphosphonates, denosumab increases BMD in men with low bone mass,[48] but it has not yet been shown to reduce fracture risk in men, except for men with nonmetastatic prostate cancer receiving androgen deprivation therapy in whom it was shown to decreased the risk of new vertebral fractures over 3 years.[49] Finally, it is worth mentioning that the Denosumab Fracture Intervention Randomized Placebo-Controlled Trial in Japanese Patients With Osteoporosis, or DIRECT trial, demonstrated that 2 years of treatment with denosumab 60 mg subcutaneously every 6 months significantly reduced the incidence of vertebral fracture compared with placebo in Japanese postmenopausal women and men with osteoporosis,[50] and the effect was maintained in a 1-year open-label extension of this trial, with a favorable benefit/risk profile.[51]

Teriparatide

In contrast to the other available antiresorptive therapies for osteoporosis, teriparatide (recombinant parathyroid hormone) is an anabolic agent that stimulates bone remodeling, preferentially increasing bone formation over resorption. In a trial of 437 men with osteoporosis randomly assigned to receive teriparatide or placebo by subcutaneous injection, teriparatide increased spine and femoral neck BMD more than placebo after 11 months of therapy.[52] The study was stopped early due to occurrence of osteosarcomas in rats, which limited the assessment of fracture reduction efficacy in these men. A 30-month follow-up analysis of the same trial showed 51% lower rate of vertebral fractures in those men previously treated with teriparatide, which was close to statistical significance.[53]

Other agents

Other agents such as romosozumab, a sclerostin monoclonal antibody, are being evaluated for the treatment of men with osteoporosis but are not currently FDA-approved for this indication.[54] In a phase III randomized trial of 245 men with osteoporosis or osteopenia and a history of fragility fracture, romosozumab increased BMD at the lumbar spine and total hip more than placebo over 12 months.[55] There were more serious cardiovascular adverse events in men receiving romosozumab versus placebo (4.9 vs 2.5%), but the difference was not statistically significant. Clinical trials for men with osteoporosis with the osteoanabolic agent abaloparatide, a parathyroid hormone–related protein analog, are not yet available.

Testosterone therapy may be appropriate in lieu of a bone-active drug for men at borderline high risk for fracture who have been diagnosed with hypogonadism (serum testosterone levels below 200 ng/dL on more than one determination, if accompanied by signs or symptoms of androgen deficiency, and for men at high risk for fracture with testosterone levels below 200 ng/dL) who have contraindications to approved pharmacologic agents for osteoporosis for men.[18]

Nonadherence to treatment

Poor adherence appears to be a major limiting factor in clinical practice. Factors associated with noncompliance include advancing age, adverse effects, pain, being unsure about BMD test results, patient health beliefs, and inadequate patient education.[56,57] Another challenge is following the specific administration requirements of oral bisphosphonates (fasting, with a full glass of water, remaining upright, and not eating for at least 30 minutes). Strategies to increase adherence include reducing administration frequency if possible, monitoring patients with bone markers and BMD testing, providing adequate instructions, practitioner feedback and support, and educational materials and sessions. More studies are needed to assess strategies aimed at increasing adherence to osteoporosis therapies in men.

CONCLUSION

In summary, therapeutic approaches to osteoporosis in men are not as well defined as in women, because antifracture efficacy data are lacking for most approved agents. Based on the currently available evidence, bisphosphonates are generally recommended as first-line pharmacotherapy in men. Despite current guidelines,[18] only approximately one-third of physicians would treat a man with osteopenia at high risk for fractures based on their FRAX score.[58] This finding emphasizes the need for continued efforts to increase awareness of osteoporosis in men to reduce undertreatment and improve patient care. Therapy needs to be individualized based on risk/benefit assessments and considering the presence of comorbid medical conditions.

As in women, osteoporosis is a major health burden in men,[59] and the incidence of osteoporotic fracture increases with advancing age. There are numerous opportunities for intervention to decrease fracture risk in men. It is important to identify and address potential factors contributing to bone loss by a careful history, physical examination, and laboratory testing to manage patients appropriately. The treatment of men with osteoporosis involves improving bone health via calcium and vitamin D supplements as well as lifestyle modification. Although these measures are important in the management of all patients, most men will likely require individualized pharmacologic therapy to adequately reduce their fracture risk. Most of the available therapies for osteoporosis in men are antiresorptive in nature. These include first-line options such as oral bisphosphonates, intravenous zoledronic acid, and subcutaneous denosumab. The only currently available osteoanabolic agent in men is teriparatide. Limitations with all these therapeutics pertain to patient compliance, antifracture efficacy at cortical sites, lack of data on sequential therapy, and concerns regarding rare but serious adverse events of long-term antiresorptive therapy.

CLINICS CARE POINTS

- Osteoporosis in men is underrecognized and undertreated. Approximately 1 in every 4 osteoporotic fractures in people older than 50 occurs in men, and the exponential increase in fracture incidence occurs approximately 1 decade later in men than in women.
- Potential contributing factors to bone loss are found in approximately 60% of men with osteoporosis and should be identified and addressed.
- Recommended strategies for identifying men at high risk of fracture are available.
- Effective agents for the treatment of men with osteoporosis should be offered to men at high risk of fracture.

DISCLOSURE

Dr D.L. Diab has nothing to disclose. Dr N.B. Watts is a speaker for Amgen and Radius.

REFERENCES

1. Osteoporosis prevention, diagnosis, and therapy. NIH Consensus Statement 2000;17(1):1–45.
2. Available at: https://www.ncbi.nlm.nih.gov/books/NBK45513/pdf/Bookshelf_NBK45513.pdf/. Accessed October 25, 2020.
3. Melton LJ 3rd. How many women have osteoporosis now? J Bone Miner Res 1995;10(2):175–7.
4. Burger H, de Laet CE, van Daele PL, et al. Risk factors for increased bone loss in an elderly population: the Rotterdam Study. Am J Epidemiol 1998;147(9):871–9.
5. Schuit SC, van der Klift M, Weel AE, et al. Fracture incidence and association with bone mineral density in elderly men and women: the Rotterdam Study. Bone 2004;34(1):195–202.
6. Available at: https://www.cdc.gov/nchs/fastats/osteoporosis.htm/. Accessed October 25, 2020.
7. Willson T, Nelson SD, Newbold J, et al. The clinical epidemiology of male osteoporosis: a review of the recent literature. Clin Epidemiol 2015;7:65–76.
8. Campion JM, Maricic MJ. Osteoporosis in men. Am Fam Physician 2003;67(7):1521–6.
9. Trombetti A, Herrmann F, Hoffmeyer P, et al. Survival and potential years of life lost after hip fracture in men and age-matched women. Osteoporos Int 2002;13(9):731–7.
10. Feldstein A, Elmer PJ, Orwoll E, et al. Bone mineral density measurement and treatment for osteoporosis in older individuals with fractures: a gap in

evidence-based practice guideline implementation. Arch Intern Med 2003; 163(18):2165–72.

11. Cosman F, de Beur SJ, LeBoff MS, et al. Clinician's Guide to Prevention and Treatment of Osteoporosis. Osteoporos Int 2014;25(10):2359–81.

12. Available at: https://www.iscd.org/official-positions/2019-iscd-official-positions-adult/. Accessed October 25, 2020.

13. Painter SE, Kleerekoper M, Camacho PM. Secondary osteoporosis: a review of the recent evidence. Endocr Pract 2006;12(4):436–45.

14. Hudec SM, Camacho PM. Secondary causes of osteoporosis. Endocr Pract 2013;19(1):120–8.

15. Stein E, Shane E. Secondary osteoporosis. Endocrinol Metab Clin North Am 2003;32(1):115–34, vii.

16. Geller JL, Hu B, Reed S, et al. Increase in bone mass after correction of vitamin D insufficiency in bisphosphonate-treated patients. Endocr Pract 2008;14(3):293–7.

17. Tannenbaum C, Clark J, Schwartzman K, et al. Yield of laboratory testing to identify secondary contributors to osteoporosis in otherwise healthy women. J Clin Endocrinol Metab 2002;87(10):4431–7.

18. Watts NB, Adler RA, Bilezikian JP, et al. Osteoporosis in men: an Endocrine Society clinical practice guideline. J Clin Endocrinol Metab 2012;97(6):1802–22.

19. Verbrugge FH, Gielen E, Milisen K, et al. Who should receive calcium and vitamin D supplementation? Age Ageing 2012;41(5):576–80.

20. Tang BM, Eslick GD, Nowson C, et al. Use of calcium or calcium in combination with vitamin D supplementation to prevent fractures and bone loss in people aged 50 years and older: a meta-analysis. Lancet 2007;370(9588):657–66.

21. Holick MF. The role of vitamin D for bone health and fracture prevention. Curr Osteoporos Rep 2006;4(3):96–102.

22. Visser M, Deeg DJ, Lips P. Low vitamin D and high parathyroid hormone levels as determinants of loss of muscle strength and muscle mass (sarcopenia): the Longitudinal Aging Study Amsterdam. J Clin Endocrinol Metab 2003;88(12):5766–72.

23. Bischoff-Ferrari HA, Staehelin HB. Importance of vitamin D and calcium at older age. Int J Vitam Nutr Res 2008;78(6):286–92.

24. Holick MF. High prevalence of vitamin D inadequacy and implications for health. Mayo Clin Proc 2006;81(3):353–73.

25. Bischoff HA, Stahelin HB, Dick W, et al. Effects of vitamin D and calcium supplementation on falls: a randomized controlled trial. J Bone Miner Res 2003;18(2): 343–51.

26. Bischoff-Ferrari HA, Dawson-Hughes B, Willett WC, et al. Effect of Vitamin D on falls: a meta-analysis. JAMA 2004;291(16):1999–2006.

27. Pfeifer M, Begerow B, Minne HW, et al. Effects of a short-term vitamin D and calcium supplementation on body sway and secondary hyperparathyroidism in elderly women. J Bone Miner Res 2000;15(6):1113–8.

28. Pfeifer M, Begerow B, Minne HW, et al. Effects of a long-term vitamin D and calcium supplementation on falls and parameters of muscle function in community-dwelling older individuals. Osteoporos Int 2009;20(2):315–22.

29. Trivedi DP, Doll R, Khaw KT. Effect of four monthly oral vitamin D3 (cholecalciferol) supplementation on fractures and mortality in men and women living in the community: randomised double blind controlled trial. BMJ 2003;326(7387):469.

30. Holick MF, Binkley NC, Bischoff-Ferrari HA, et al. Evaluation, treatment, and prevention of vitamin D deficiency: an Endocrine Society clinical practice guideline. J Clin Endocrinol Metab 2011;96(7):1911–30.

31. Bischoff-Ferrari HA. Optimal serum 25-hydroxyvitamin D levels for multiple health outcomes. Adv Exp Med Biol 2008;624:55–71.
32. Holick MF, Binkley NC, Bischoff-Ferrari HA, et al. Guidelines for preventing and treating vitamin D deficiency and insufficiency revisited. J Clin Endocrinol Metab 2012;97(4):1153–8.
33. Ebeling PR. Osteoporosis in men. Curr Opin Rheumatol 2013;25(4):542–52.
34. Watts NB. Osteoporosis in men. Endocr Pract 2013;19(5):834–8.
35. Orwoll E, Ettinger M, Weiss S, et al. Alendronate for the treatment of osteoporosis in men. N Engl J Med 2000;343(9):604–10.
36. Sawka AM, Papaioannou A, Adachi JD, et al. Does alendronate reduce the risk of fracture in men? A meta-analysis incorporating prior knowledge of anti-fracture efficacy in women. BMC Musculoskelet Disord 2005;6:39.
37. Xu Z. Alendronate for the treatment of osteoporosis in men: a meta-analysis of randomized controlled trials. Am J Ther 2017;24(2):e130–8.
38. Stoch SA, Saag KG, Greenwald M, et al. Once-weekly oral alendronate 70 mg in patients with glucocorticoid-induced bone loss: a 12-month randomized, placebo-controlled clinical trial. J Rheumatol 2009;36(8):1705–14.
39. Greenspan SL, Nelson JB, Trump DL, et al. Effect of once-weekly oral alendronate on bone loss in men receiving androgen deprivation therapy for prostate cancer: a randomized trial. Ann Intern Med 2007;146(6):416–24.
40. Ringe JD, Faber H, Farahmand P, et al. Efficacy of risedronate in men with primary and secondary osteoporosis: results of a 1-year study. Rheumatol Int 2006;26(5):427–31.
41. Ringe JD, Farahmand P, Faber H, et al. Sustained efficacy of risedronate in men with primary and secondary osteoporosis: results of a 2-year study. Rheumatol Int 2009;29(3):311–5.
42. Boonen S, Orwoll ES, Wenderoth D, et al. Once-weekly risedronate in men with osteoporosis: results of a 2-year, placebo-controlled, double-blind, multicenter study. J Bone Miner Res 2009;24(4):719–25.
43. Boonen S, Reginster JY, Kaufman JM, et al. Fracture risk and zoledronic acid therapy in men with osteoporosis. N Engl J Med 2012;367(18):1714–23.
44. Nayak S, Greenspan SL. Osteoporosis treatment efficacy for men: a systematic review and meta-analysis. J Am Geriatr Soc 2017;65(3):490–5.
45. Sim Ie W, Ebeling PR. Treatment of osteoporosis in men with bisphosphonates: rationale and latest evidence. Ther Adv Musculoskelet Dis 2013;5(5):259–67.
46. Adler RA. Update on osteoporosis in men. Best Pract Res Clin Endocrinol Metab 2018;32(5):759–72.
47. Kharazmi M, Hallberg P, Michaëlsson K. Gender related difference in the risk of bisphosphonate associated atypical femoral fracture and osteonecrosis of the jaw. Ann Rheum Dis 2014;73(8):1594.
48. Orwoll E, Teglbjærg CS, Langdahl BL, et al. A randomized, placebo-controlled study of the effects of denosumab for the treatment of men with low bone mineral density. J Clin Endocrinol Metab 2012;97(9):3161–9.
49. Smith MR, Egerdie B, Hernández Toriz N, et al. Denosumab in men receiving androgen-deprivation therapy for prostate cancer. N Engl J Med 2009;361(8):745–55.
50. Nakamura T, Matsumoto T, Sugimoto T, et al. Clinical Trials Express: fracture risk reduction with denosumab in Japanese postmenopausal women and men with osteoporosis: denosumab fracture intervention randomized placebo controlled trial (DIRECT). J Clin Endocrinol Metab 2014;99(7):2599–607.

51. Sugimoto T, Matsumoto T, Hosoi T, et al. Three-year denosumab treatment in postmenopausal Japanese women and men with osteoporosis: results from a 1-year open-label extension of the Denosumab Fracture Intervention Randomized Placebo Controlled Trial (DIRECT). Osteoporos Int 2015;26(2):765–74.

52. Orwoll ES, Scheele WH, Paul S, et al. The effect of teriparatide [human parathyroid hormone (1-34)] therapy on bone density in men with osteoporosis. J Bone Miner Res 2003;18(1):9–17.

53. Kaufman JM, Orwoll E, Goemaere S, et al. Teriparatide effects on vertebral fractures and bone mineral density in men with osteoporosis: treatment and discontinuation of therapy. Osteoporos Int 2005;16(5):510–6.

54. Gennari L, Bilezikian JP. New and developing pharmacotherapy for osteoporosis in men. Expert Opin Pharmacother 2018;19(3):253–64.

55. Lewiecki EM, Blicharski T, Goemaere S, et al. A Phase III randomized placebo-controlled trial to evaluate efficacy and safety of romosozumab in men with osteoporosis. J Clin Endocrinol Metab 2018;103(9):3183–93.

56. Papaioannou A, Kennedy CC, Dolovich L, et al. Patient adherence to osteoporosis medications: problems, consequences and management strategies. Drugs Aging 2007;24(1):37–55.

57. Gold DT, Silverman S. Review of adherence to medications for the treatment of osteoporosis. Curr Osteoporos Rep 2006;4(1):21–7.

58. Papaleontiou M, Choksi P, Reyes-Gastelum D. Practice patterns in the treatment of male osteoporosis. Endocr Pract 2019;25(10):1077–8.

59. Gennari L, Bilezikian JP. Osteoporosis in men. Endocrinol Metab Clin North Am 2007;36(2):399–419.

Glucocorticoid- and Transplantation-Induced Osteoporosis

Guido Zavatta, MD[a,b], Bart L. Clarke, MD[a],*

KEYWORDS

- Glucocorticoids • Corticosteroids • Glucocorticoid-induced osteoporosis
- Transplant-induced osteoporosis • Osteoporosis • Fracture • BMD • Treatment

KEY POINTS

- Reduced bone formation due to osteoblast damage, continued bone resorption, and reduced skeletal sensing of biomechanical forces due to osteocyte apoptosis, are the main pathophysiological mechanisms causing glucocorticoid-induced osteoporosis (GIOP).
- Bone microarchitecture is severely compromised in GIOP, whereas areal bone mineral density (BMD) may be less affected.
- There does not appear to be a threshold dose of cumulative glucocorticoid therapy that identifies patients who will fracture, although chronic doses of prednisone equivalent greater than 7.5 mg per day are associated with a high incidence of fragility fractures.
- Transplantation-induced osteoporosis encompasses a broad range of unique pathogenetic features depending on end-stage organ disease and the transplanted organ, which have implications for the type and timing of osteoporotic treatment.

INTRODUCTION

Excess endogenous or exogenous glucocorticoids increase fracture risk. Even mild adrenal overproduction of cortisol is associated with increased risk of vertebral fracture.[1] Glucocorticoids used to treat a variety of chronic medical conditions increase the risk of bone loss and fracture. In the United States, as many as 2.5 million patients (1% of the population 20 years of age or older) routinely receive oral glucocorticoid therapy, thereby making glucocorticoid-induced osteoporosis the most frequent cause of secondary osteoporosis.

[a] Mayo Clinic E18-A, 200 1st Street Southwest, Rochester, MN 55905, USA; [b] Division of Endocrinology and Diabetes Prevention and Care, IRCCS Azienda Ospedaliero-Universitaria di Bologna, Department of Medical and Surgical Sciences (DIMEC), Alma Mater Studiorum, University of Bologna, Policlinico di S. Orsola - Padiglione 11, Via Massarenti 9, Bologna 40138, Italy
* Corresponding author.
E-mail address: clarke.bart@mayo.edu

Endocrinol Metab Clin N Am 50 (2021) 251–273
https://doi.org/10.1016/j.ecl.2021.03.002
0889-8529/21/© 2021 Elsevier Inc. All rights reserved.

Transplantation-induced osteoporosis is a complex metabolic bone disorder due in part to the effects of chronic glucocorticoid therapy. The pathophysiology of transplantation-induced osteoporosis varies depending on the type of end-stage organ disease and transplanted organ, so that therapeutic decisions are more complicated. There are few long-term fracture data in treated transplant populations, although clinical experience suggests a persistent burden of clinical fractures predicted in part by bone mineral density (BMD).

GLUCOCORTICOID-INDUCED OSTEOPOROSIS
Pathophysiology of Glucocorticoid-induced Osteoporosis

Multiple factors are involved in glucocorticoid-induced bone loss (**Fig. 1**). Dose, duration, and route of administration of glucocorticoids should all be considered when assessing potential for damage to bone.

The isoenzymes 11-beta-hydroxysteroid dehydrogenase type 1 (11β-HSD1) and type 2 (11β-HSD2) affect cortisol levels in the blood. 11β-HSD1 catalyzes the conversion of inactive cortisone into active cortisol. 11β-HSD2 does the opposite. Conversion of cortisol and related biologically active glucocorticoids into inactive cortisone protects bone cells and the skeleton. In vitro activity of 11β-HSD1 increases with age, dose, and duration of glucocorticoid treatment,[2] and leads to greater cortisol exposure and higher fragility fracture rates, especially in elderly individuals.[3,4]

When glucocorticoids are used therapeutically, deterioration of both BMD and quality of bone occurs as a result of multiple effects on bone resorption and bone formation. A transient increase in bone resorption over the first 12 to 18 months after starting therapy is followed by maintenance of normal bone resorption and persistently reduced bone formation over as many years as therapy is continued. Decreased

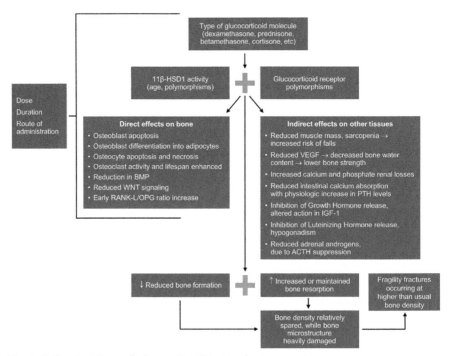

Fig. 1. Pathophysiology of glucocorticoid-induced osteoporosis.

bone formation and maintained normal bone resorption are thought to be the key pathogenetic mechanisms causing bone loss, worsening of bone strength, and development of fractures over time. Osteoblast and osteocyte apoptosis increase with persistent glucocorticoid excess, whereas osteoclast recruitment increases during early exposure.

Glucocorticoids decrease intestinal calcium absorption by disrupting both active transport of calcium in the gut[5] and vitamin D metabolism.[6] As a result, serum parathyroid hormone (PTH) levels may increase, often within the physiologic range. Glucocorticoids stimulate renal calcium[7] and phosphate[8] urinary excretion,[7] thereby further worsening negative mineral balance. Glucocorticoids may also decrease the secretion of growth hormone, gonadotropins, and adrenocorticotropic hormone, which in turn lowers serum insulinlike growth factor (IGF)-1, estrogens, and both gonadal and adrenal androgens. In addition, glucocorticoids may directly reduce IGF-1 and IGF1-binding protein (IGF-BP) levels.[9]

Reduction of blood flow through bone associated with glucocorticoid suppression of VEGF production[10] may lead to dehydration of bone, which has been associated with reduction in bone strength.[3] In mice, it appears that bone water content and crystallinity, a measure of hydroxyapatite crystal size, may be impaired due to aging and glucocorticoid dose, thus causing an alteration in the load-bearing properties of bone.[10]

The result of this multiplicity of changes is a generalized catabolic state in which bone loss, adverse changes in bone and muscle microarchitecture and strength, muscle loss (sarcopenia), and fractures are more likely to occur.[11]

At the molecular level, the RANKL (receptor activator of nuclear factor-kB ligand)-RANK-OPG (osteoprotegerin) system is significantly affected. RANKL is secreted by osteoblasts and osteocytes and interacts with its receptor RANK on osteoclasts and osteoclast precursors to cause osteoclast recruitment, activation, and bone loss. OPG is produced by osteoblasts and acts as a decoy receptor for RANKL, preventing it from binding to RANK on osteoclasts. In GIOP, initially higher levels of RANKL are observed, along with reduced levels of OPG,[12] thereby promoting the activation of osteoclasts. Subsequently, RANKL expression declines over time, apparently secondary to depletion of osteoblasts.

Although its impact remains to be assessed, low glucocorticoid doses appear to preserve autophagy, and thereby preserve normal osteoblast functionality. High glucocorticoid doses suppress autophagy, and favor osteoblast apoptosis.[13]

Schepper and colleagues[14] recently reported a direct link between gut microbiota and trabecular bone loss in glucocorticoid-treated mice. Wide-spectrum antibiotics or the probiotic *Lactobacillus reuteri* were able to prevent trabecular bone loss during glucocorticoid therapy. Preservation of intestinal barrier function blunted bone loss as well. Transplanting fecal material from glucocorticoid-treated mice into glucocorticoid treatment-naïve mice resulted in bone loss. These findings suggested that changes in microbiota composition and intestinal permeability caused by glucocorticoid treatment may also cause bone loss.

Alteration in Bone Density and Quality

GIOP is characterized by deterioration of bone microarchitecture as well as loss of bone mass. Worsening of bone microarchitecture before significant bone loss may explain the early increase in fracture risk without preceding bone loss detected by dual-energy x-ray absorptiometry (DXA). Trabecular bone is more affected by glucocorticoids than cortical bone, putatively because of its greater metabolic activity and surface area.

Trabecular bone score (TBS) has been shown to predict fracture risk independently of DXA during glucocorticoid therapy, and is currently being used clinically. Proprietary software (TBS Insight; Medimaps, Meriganc, France) is used to conduct a gray-level texture assessment of lumbar spine DXA images to assess the skeletal micro-architecture. Lower TBS values are observed in women with recent fractures, or in women without fractures treated with glucocorticoids. TBS may be able to refine fracture risk prediction by DXA in glucocorticoid-treated patients, and it has recently been included in the FRAX algorithm.[15]

High-resolution peripheral quantitative computed tomography (HRpQCT) is able to precisely assess trabecular and cortical structure of bone. In a multicenter study[16] of men with GIOP, HRpQCT-derived BMD was able to identify patients with prevalent vertebral fractures, whereas DXA could not. When bone microstructure is evaluated by HRpQCT, finite element analysis can be used to predict bone strength.

Fractures

Vertebral fractures are the most common fractures reported in patients with GIOP. Fracture risk is significantly increased as early as 3 months after the start of glucocorticoid therapy[17] and peaks at approximately 12 months.[18] Fracture incidence decreases rapidly after cessation of corticosteroids regardless of the preceding cumulative dose. The reduction in fracture risk can be detected as early as 3 to 12 months after the discontinuation of glucocorticoids. The greater the daily dose of glucocorticoid, the higher the fracture risk. In the UK General Practice Research Database, patients receiving prednisolone equivalent greater than 7.5 mg/d had more than twofold increased risk of vertebral or hip fractures compared with those taking less than 2.5 mg/d. Patients receiving prednisolone 2.5 to 7.5 mg/d had at least a 50% increase in risk of vertebral and hip fractures compared with those taking less than 2.5 mg/d.[17] Prednisolone equivalent doses as low as 2.5 mg/d have been associated with a relative risk of 1.17 (95% confidence interval [CI] 1.10–1.25) for nonvertebral fractures and 1.55 (95% CI 1.20–2.01) for vertebral fractures.[19] These fractures may be due to incompletely suppressed systemic inflammation due underlying disease. Low glucocorticoid doses are commonly used in rheumatologic disorders and transplant recipients.

Recent work has revealed an increased risk of fracture in patients with adrenal adenomas overproducing cortisol (HR 1.24; 95% CI 1.04–1.48), regardless of the threshold used for dexamethasone suppression. These findings were interpreted as indicating that even undiagnosed abnormal cortisol secretion by adrenal adenomas may be harmful to the skeleton.[20]

Intermittent use of high-dose oral glucocorticoids (>15 mg/d) has been associated with an increase in fragility fractures, but not specifically hip fractures, with cumulative exposure of less than 1 g. When cumulative exposure is higher, especially greater than 5 g, a substantial increase in fracture risk is observed despite the intermittent exposure, similar to what is observed during continuous treatment.[21]

The country-specific fracture risk algorithm FRAX is used to estimate 10-year absolute fracture risk. FRAX estimates are most accurate when doses of glucocorticoids range between 2.5 to 7.5 mg/d. However, if daily doses are less than or more than these limits, FRAX is likely to underestimate or overestimate fracture risk, respectively. Therefore, for doses less than 2.5 mg/d, FRAX risk should be adjusted downward by 20%, whereas if doses exceed 7.5 mg daily, FRAX risk should be adjusted upward by 15%.[22]

Bone Turnover Markers in Glucocorticoid-induced Osteoporosis

Bone turnover markers (BTMs) may be useful in patients treated with glucocorticoids to determine bone turnover, and thereby guide treatment with antiresorptive or anabolic agents. N-terminal propeptide of type 1 collagen (P1NP) and bone-specific alkaline phosphatase (BSAP) are serum markers of osteoblast activity and bone formation that may be decreased by glucocorticoid treatment. Serum osteocalcin reflects both bone formation and bone resorption. Serum β-CTx-telopeptide (CTx) is associated with osteoclast resorption activity, which may be increased during early glucocorticoid treatment. Osteocalcin is generally suppressed during glucocorticoid overproduction or treatment, and this BTM has been proposed as a bone turnover marker useful in endogenous Cushing syndrome.[23] Serum sclerostin is usually decreased in patients treated with glucocorticoids due to reduced osteocyte number and function.[24]

Treatment

Optimization of calcium intake through diet and/or supplements, and maintenance of adequate serum levels of 25-hydroxyvitamin D (>30 ng/mL) are necessary but not sufficient to prevent bone loss or fractures during glucocorticoid therapy. Recommended calcium intake varies in different guidelines, but the 2011 Institute of Medicine recommended daily allowance (RDA) was 1200 mg through diet and supplements, with the cholecalciferol RDA 600 to 800 IU.

Effective treatments for glucocorticoid-induced osteoporosis and their effects on bone density are shown in **Table 1**. Food and Drug Administration–approved treatments for GIOP based on bone density protection only include oral alendronate 5 mg/d for men and premenopausal women, and 10 mg/d for postmenopausal women not receiving estrogen therapy, oral risedronate 5 mg/d, subcutaneously injected teriparatide 20 μg/d, intravenous zoledronic acid 5 mg once each year, and subcutaneously injected denosumab 60 mg every 6 months. Duration of therapy in most clinical trials was up to 2 years, but these agents may be used longer if clinically indicated. Although commonly prescribed in clinical practice, weekly and monthly formulations of oral bisphosphonates have not been approved specifically for the treatment of GIOP. None of the GIOP treatment trials were powered to assess fracture reduction.

Abaloparatide, a PTH-related protein–related analogue, has not yet been evaluated in clinical trials in GIOP. A recent study of abaloparatide in ovariectomized glucocorticoid-treated rabbits has shown promising results.[25] Abaloparatide benefitted both cortical and trabecular bone properties, as well as femoral strength.

No data are yet available regarding the potential benefit of the anti-sclerostin antibody romosozumab in GIOP.

TRANSPLANTATION-INDUCED OSTEOPOROSIS

Transplantation-induced osteoporosis may be considered as a special subtype of GIOP. However, as opposed to glucocorticoid treatment, which may be short-term, of variable length, or given on an intermittent schedule by different routes, and titrated as rapidly as possible to the lowest effective dose to minimize adverse effects, transplantation is a chronic nonreversible condition in which glucocorticoid therapy is usually given in stable low doses, with additional factors contributing to bone damage. End-stage organ disease is present in all patients before transplantation, and treatments and complications from these various diseases usually has a significant impact on the skeleton. In pretransplant patients, identification of risk factors for bone loss should be part of the pretransplant evaluation (**Table 2**).

All previously published studies investigating bone disease in transplant populations, regardless of the organ, are limited in size and none of them have robust data regarding the effectiveness of osteoporosis medications in reducing fracture risk. In

Table 1
Major randomized clinical trials in glucocorticoid-induced osteoporosis

First Author, year	Active Drug	Duration	Placebo/Control Drug	Age (y)	F %	GC-Initiating	GC-Continuing	Prednisone-Equivalent Dose (mg)	Lumbar Spine BMD (% change)	Femoral Neck BMD (% change)	Total Hip BMD (% change)	Fractures
Saag et al,[51] 1998	ALN 10 mg/d	48 wk	800–1000 Ca + 250–500 U Vit D3	55 ± 15	77		✓	10	2.9 vs −0.4	1 vs −1.2	0.7 vs −0.07	NA
Wallach et al,[52] 2000	RIS 5 mg/d	12 mo	1000 Ca + 400 U Vit D3	59.3 ± 13.2	64		✓	13 ± 1	1.9 vs −1.0	1.3 vs −1.5	NA	−70% vs placebo
Adachi et al,[53] 2001	ALN 10 mg/d	24 mo	800–1000 Ca + 250–500 U Vit D3	53 ± 15	72		✓	17 ± 18	3.9 vs −0.8	0.61 vs −2.93	2.69 vs 1.57	−89% vs placebo
de Nijs et al,[54] 2006	ALN 10 mg/d	18 mo	alfacalcidol 1 μg/d	60 ± 14	60	✓		23 ± 20	2.1 vs −1.9	1.4 vs −2.0	0.8 vs 2.2	Similar
Saag et al,[55] 2007	TERIP 20 μg/d	18 mo	ALN 10 mg/d	56.1 ± 13.4	80		✓	7.5	7.2 vs 3.4	NA	3.8 vs 2.4	Reduced vertebral fractures
Saag et al,[56] 2009	TERIP 20 μg/d	36 mo	ALN 10 mg/d	56.1 ± 13.4	80		✓	7.5	11.0 vs 5.3	6.3 vs 3.4	5.2 vs 2.7	−78% vertebral fractures
Stoch et al,[57] 2009	ALN 70 mg/wk	12 mo	1000 Ca + 400 U Vit D3	51.9 ± 14.4	61		✓	16.5 (start)-10.3(end)	2.45 vs −0.47	0.41% vs 0.08 (NS)	0.75 vs 0.44	NA
Mok et al,[58] 2011	RALOX 60 mg/d	12 mo	1000 Ca + calcitriol 0.25 μg/d (on top)	55.4 ± 7.8	100		✓	6.7 ± 5.9	1.3 vs −0.9	NS	1.0 vs 0.8	NA

Study	Drug	Duration	Comparator	Age	%		GC	Spine	Total hip	Femoral neck	Fracture
Hakala et al,[59] 2012	IBAN 150 mg/mo	12 mo	1000 Ca + 800 U Vit D3	64 ± 8	100	✓	6.7 ± 2.7	3.2 vs −0.1	2.0 vs −0.6	1.2 vs −0.7	NA
Sambrook et al,[60] 2012	ZOL 5 mg IV q year	12 mo	RIS 5 mg/d	59 ± 16	0	✓	18.9 ± 19.4	2.46 vs −0.24	1.37 vs −0.02 (NS)	1.10 vs 0.39	NA
Sambrook et al,[60] 2012	ZOL 5 mg IV q year	12 mo	RIS 5 mg/d	56 ± 13	0	✓	13.3 ± 7.9	4.69 vs 3.27	1.31 vs 0.38 (NS)	1.82 vs 0.18	NA
Gluer et al,[61] 2012	TERIP 20 μg/d	18 mo	RIS 35 mg/wk	57.5 ± 12.8	0	✓	8.8	16.3 vs 3.8 (L1-L3 QCT BMD)	NA	NA	NA
Saag et al,[62] 2018	DEN 60 mg twice/y	12 mo	RIS 5 mg/d	67.5 ± 10.1	64	✓	12.3	3.8 vs 0.8	0.9 vs −0.2	1.7 vs 0.2	NA
Saag et al,[62] 2018	DEN 60 mg twice/y	12 mo	RIS 5 mg/d	61.5 ± 11.6	72	✓	16.6	4.4 vs 2.3	1.6 vs 0.6	2.1 vs 0.6	NA
Saag et al,[63] 2019	DEN 60 mg twice/year	24 mo	RIS 5 mg/d	67.5 ± 10.1	64	✓	12.3	6.2 vs 1.7	1.5 vs −0.9	3.1 vs 0.0	Similar
Saag et al,[63] 2019	DEN 60 mg twice/year	24 mo	RIS 5 mg/d	61.5 ± 11.6	72	✓	16.6	6.4 vs 3.2	2.2 vs 0.4	2.9 vs 0.5	Similar

Abbreviations: ALN, alendronate; BMD, bone mineral density; Ca, calcium carbonate supplements; DEN, denosumab; F, female; GC, glucocorticoid; IBAN, ibandronate; IV, intravenous; NA, not available; NS, non-significant; RALOX, raloxifene; q, every; QCT, quantitative computed tomography; RIS, risedronate; TERIP, teriparatide; Vit D3, Vitamin D3; ZOL, zoledronic acid.

Table 2
Pre- and Post-transplant risk factors for bone loss or fractures before and after solid organ or stem-cell transplantation

Pre-transplant risk factors associated with bone loss or fractures before and after solid organ or stem-cell transplantation.

Age	Prior vertebral fractures
Low BMI	Low pre-transplant BMD
Hypogonadism	Low 25-OH vitamin D
Tobacco use	Pancreatic insufficiency (cystic fibrosis)
Alcohol abuse	Pre-transplant diabetes
Prolonged immobilization	Pre-transplant dialysis
Secondary hyperparathyroidism	Cholestatic liver disease
Chronic kidney disease	High-dose chemotherapy
Medications (glucocorticoids)	Total body irradiation
Congestive heart failure	Secondary causes of osteoporosis

Post-transplant risk factors associated with bone loss or fractures after solid organ or stem-cell transplantation.

Female Gender	High-dose glucocorticoids
Hyperparathyroidism	Organ rejections
Duration of immobilization after transplantation	Gonadal hormone status
Nonsteroidal immunosuppressants (cyclosporine, tacrolimus)	Low turnover or Adynamic bone disease
Hyperphosphaturia/Hypophosphatemia	Osteomalacia

Abbreviations: BMD, bone mineral density; BMI, body mass index.

fact, most studies only describe effects on BMD or BTMs. Calcium and vitamin D supplementation is typically recommended based on the GIOP recommendations. Common challenges in clinical practice are how to care for patients younger than 50 years, how to treat women of child-bearing potential with very low BMD and/or multiple fractures, and how best to treat older patients with comorbidities that limit therapeutic choices.

Nonsteroidal Immunosuppressants

Nonsteroidal immunosuppressants are incorporated into posttransplantation regimens to reduce or, in some cases, eliminate long-term glucocorticoid therapy, and thereby minimize skeletal and other adverse effects. Cyclosporine and tacrolimus are calcineurin inhibitors commonly used, with their impact on human bone health still not clear. Older studies in rats showed negative effects,[26] but evidence in humans has been variable, and studies have not consistently shown adverse effects.

Evidence regarding other immunosuppressants is limited. Compared with cyclosporine, rapamycin (sirolimus) is associated with lower serum osteocalcin and urinary NTx-telopeptide in renal transplant patients.[27] One study showed that rapamycin may negatively affect differentiating osteoblasts by downregulating *Runx2*, thereby leading to lower bone formation and mineralization capacity.[28] However, other studies have suggested that rapamycin may have a potential anti-aging effect on bone.[29] The impacts of azathioprine and mycophenolate mofetil are thought to be minimal, if any, whereas the effect of daclizumab is unknown.

Table 3
Bone status before transplantation

Evidence	End-Organ Disease	BMD	Fractures
Majumdar et al,[31] 2012	Congestive heart failure	40% osteoporosis	30% increase in major fractures, independent of traditional risk factors and BMD.
Monegal et al,[32] 2001	End-stage liver disease	51% osteopenia, 24% osteoporosis. Patients with DXA criteria for osteoporosis at higher risk of fractures after OLT (OR 5.6, 95% CI 1.31–24.53).	22% of patients have prevalent vertebral fractures. BMD not correlated with prevalent vertebral fractures.
Alem et al,[33] 2000	Stage 5 chronic kidney disease on hemodialysis	NR[a]	Incidence of hip fracture is approximately fourfold higher compared with the general population, and increases with age.
Schulte et al,[34] 2000	Hematological malignancies	24% osteopenia, 4% osteoporosis.	NR
Tschopp et al,[35] 2002	Chronic respiratory failure	T score < −1.0 in approximately 60% of patients. Strong association with low BMI.	NR
Resnick et al,[36] 2010	Severe bowel disease (81% with primary intestinal disease or visceral vascular thrombosis)	41.5% osteopenia, 35.9% osteoporosis.	6%

Abbreviations: BMD, bone mineral density; CI, confidence interval; DXA, dual-energy x-ray absorptiometry; NR, not reported; OLT, orthotopic liver transplant; OR, odds-ratio.

[a] BMD by DXA is not a reliable indicator of fracture risk in patients with end-stage renal disease (ESRD) as opposed to patients without ESRD.

Pretransplant Bone Loss Due to End-Organ Disease

Preexisting bone disease is a major determinant of the subsequent impact of transplantation on the skeleton.[30] Before transplantation, prevalence of osteoporosis is variable and partially dependent on the underlying end-organ disease (**Table 3**) and general health of the patient. Osteoporosis has been described in up to 40% of patients with congestive heart failure.[31] Osteoporosis and fractures are reported in 11% to 52% of patients with end-stage liver disease.[30,32] Patients with stage 5 chronic kidney disease on hemodialysis have a fourfold increased risk of hip fractures compared with age- and sex-matched controls from the general population.[33] Patients undergoing stem-cell transplantation (SCT) are exposed to high-dose glucocorticoids and chemotherapeutic agents, with low BMD affecting almost a third of these patients.[30,34] In chronic respiratory failure, low BMD may affect up to 61% of affected individuals.[35] Older age and duration of parenteral nutrition are correlated with osteoporosis in approximately 36% of candidates for intestinal transplantation.[36] Improved survival rates after transplantation require that measures for primary and secondary fracture prevention be implemented in patients with end-stage organ disease who may be candidates for solid organ transplantation or SCT. **Table 2** summarizes risk factors for posttransplantation bone loss.

Heart Transplantation

The first 12 months posttransplant is the most critical period for bone loss in patients undergoing heart transplantation. Trabecular bone loss seems to be greater than cortical bone loss in the first 6 months, whereas cortical bone is more affected in the subsequent 6 months.[37] Thereafter, BMD may stabilize or partially recover with maintenance doses of glucocorticoids. Early studies reported decreases in BMD that were variable, ranging from 6% to 11% at both the lumbar spine and hip during the first year. Prevalent vertebral fractures were as high as 40%, with maximum incidence in the first year after transplant.[30] A recent study did not report such high numbers of incident fractures, showing only 12% incidence of new vertebral fractures, without other peripheral fractures.[38] Lumbar spine BMD may progressively increase with adequate calcium and vitamin D for up to 10 years after cardiac transplantation, rising above baseline at transplantation, whereas proximal femoral BMD tends to remain stable below pretransplant values.[39] Fractures steadily increase for up to 4 years after transplantation, from 21% to 32%. An overview of treatment trials in heart transplant recipients is shown in **Table 4**.

Liver Transplantation

Liver transplant patients commonly sustain significant bone loss, as well as rib and vertebral fractures, within the first 6 to 12 months after transplantation. Fractures occurred in 21% of patients in the first year and 33% in the fourth year following transplantation.[40] Patients with prior cholestatic liver disease are at higher risk of developing subsequent fractures.[41] Smaller amounts of bone loss have been reported in more recent studies. A recent longitudinal study in untreated patients revealed persistently low bone density for up to 15 years after transplantation,[42] thus pointing out significant undertreatment of liver transplantation osteoporosis. Treatment trials to prevent bone loss in liver transplant recipients are shown in **Table 5**. Bisphosphonates are able to increase lumbar spine BMD, whereas hip BMD is less affected.[43] A recent small retrospective study showed denosumab to significantly improve lumbar spine T-scores.[44] A prospective study of liver transplant patients treated with denosumab is currently ongoing (ClinicalTrials.gov Identifier: NCT04231682), with results expected in 2025.

Kidney Transplantation

Rates of bone loss in kidney transplant recipients appear to be greatest in the first 6 to 18 months.[45] As opposed to heart or liver transplant patients, fractures are more likely to occur at appendicular sites, including the femur, ankles, long bones, and feet, rather than axial sites. Persistent hyperparathyroidism after transplantation leads to long-term cortical and trabecular bone loss. Because low-turnover or adynamic bone disease might persist even with increased serum parathyroid hormone levels after transplantation, bone biopsy is recommended to discriminate between high or low bone turnover. As a consequence, decisions regarding the best therapeutic options should not be based solely on DXA or the parathyroid hormone level. Both intravenous and oral bisphosphonates have been used with positive outcomes on BMD (**Table 6**), but adynamic bone disease remains a concern with use of antiresorptive agents.

Table 4
Therapies for Reducing Bone Loss in Heart Transplantation, in addition to Calcium or Vitamin D

Molecule	Duration	Age	F%	Dose	Route of Administration	Lumbar Spine BMD (% change)	Femoral Neck BMD (% change)	Total Hip BMD (% change)	Fractures/Comments
Calcidiol[64] (Delgado, 1997)	18 mo	51.5 ± 2.9	15.4	32,000 U weekly	Oral	4.9	NA	NA	No vertebral fractures (13 patients) vs etidronate (3/14) or calcitonin (4/13)
Pamidronate + etidronate[65] (Shane, 1998)	12 mo	NA	NA	Pamidronate 60 mg IV within 2 wk followed by cyclic oral Etidronate (14 consecutive days every 3 mo)	IV + Oral	−0.9	−2.7	NA	Less bone loss and fewer fractures (3/18) than those treated with calcium and vitamin D (18/52)
Calcitriol[66] (Sambrook, 2000)	24 mo	NA	NA	0.5–0.75 µg/d	Oral	−2.7	−5	NA	Less bone loss and fewer vertebral fractures compared with calcium alone
Calcitonin + calcitriol[67] (Bianda,2000)	18 mo	54 ± 1	8.3	200 U + 0.5 µg daily	Nasal Calcitonin	−6.5	−6.1	NA	1 vertebral fracture (out of 12 patients)
Pamidronate[67] (Bianda, 2000)	18 mo	51 ± 3	7.1	0.5 mg/kg every 3 mo	IV	−3.8	−3.0	NA	NA
Pamidronate[68] (Krieg, 2001)	36 mo	46 ± 4	9.0	60 mg every 3 mo	IV	14.3	NS	NA	−7.8% loss at femoral neck with placebo; no clinical fractures occurred
Clodronate[69] (Ippoliti, 2003)	12 mo	5 0 ± 17	9.4	1600 mg/d	Oral	11.7	NA	NA	0% fractures vs 9.3% in the placebo group

(continued on next page)

Table 4
(continued)

Molecule	Duration	Age	F%	Dose	Route of Administration	Lumbar Spine BMD (% change)	Femoral Neck BMD (% change)	Total Hip BMD (% change)	Fractures/Comments
Alendronate[70] (Shane, 2004)	12 mo	54 ± 11	15%	10 mg/d	Oral	−0.7	−1.7	−1.5	BMD % changes significant vs calcitriol; no difference in fractures
Ibandronate[71] (Fahrleitner-Pammer, 2009)	12 mo	45 ± 6	NA	2 mg every 3 mo	IV	Unchanged (vs −25)	Unchanged (vs −23)	NA	Absolute and relative vertebral fracture risk reduction of 40% and 75%, respectively
Weekly alendronate or risedronate[72] (Lange, 2017)	24 mo	54 ± 11	24.2	70 mg weekly/ 35 mg weekly	Oral	NS	NA	NS	No fractures during follow-up

Abbreviations: BMD, bone mineral density; F, female; IV, intravenous; NA, not available; NS, nonsignificant.

Table 5
Therapies for Reducing Bone Loss in Liver Transplantation, in addition to Calcium or Vitamin D

Molecule	Duration	Age	F%	Dose	Route of Administration	Lumbar Spine BMD (% change)	Femoral Neck BMD (% change)	Total Hip BMD (% change)	Fractures/Comments
Zoledronate[73] (Crawford, 2006)	12 mo	47.4 ± 9.7	18.8	4 mg at m 0, 1, 3, 6, 9	IV	NS vs placebo	NS vs placebo	+2.4% vs placebo	Similar
Pamidronate[74] (Pennisi, 2006)	12 mo	54.7 ± 10.0	28.4	30 mg every 3 mo	IV	T-score improvement (+1.07)	T-score decrease (−0.2)	NA	Fewer clinical fractures in treatment group (1 vs 3)
Alendronate + Calcitriol[75] (Atamaz, 2006)	12 mo	42.6 ± 11.4	18.6	70 mg weekly + 0.50 µg daily	Oral	Increase, not specified	Increase, not specified	Increase, not specified	No fractures
Zoledronate[76] (Bodingbauer, 2007)	12 mo	52 ± 8.2	25.5	4 mg at mo 0, 1, 2, 3, 4, 5, 6, 9, 12	IV	Stable	Stable	NA	Significant reduction of fractures
Pamidronate[77] (Monegal, 2009)	12 mo	52.8 ± 11.20	12.5	90 mg at baseline and 3 mo	IV	2.9	−3.2 (NS)	NA	Similar
Ibandronate[78] (Kaemmerer, 2010)	24 mo	51.5 ± 14.0	58.8	2 mg every 3 mo	IV	NS	NS	NA	Fewer clinical fractures (7% vs 25%)
Risedronate[79] (Guadalix, 2011)	12 mo	57.9 ± 6.5	29	35 mg weekly	Oral	~5%	NS	NS	10% morphometric vertebral fractures vs 21% in control (NS)

(continued on next page)

Table 5
(continued)

Molecule	Duration	Age	F%	Dose	Route of Administration	Lumbar Spine BMD (% change)	Femoral Neck BMD (% change)	Total Hip BMD (% change)	Fractures/ Comments
Zoledronate[80] (Shane, 2012)	12 mo	55 ± 8	27	5 mg within 30 d of transplantation	IV	2.0%	NS	NS	NS
Denosumab[44] (Brunova, 2018)	1.65 ± 0.7 y	NA	NA	60 mg every 6 mo	SC	11.4 ± 7.7	NA	NS (based only on T-scores of proximal femur)	NA

Abbreviations: BMD, bone mineral density; F, female; IV, intravenous; NA, not available; NS, nonsignificant.

Table 6
Therapies for Reducing Bone Loss in Kidney Transplantation, in addition to Calcium or Vitamin D

Molecule	Duration	Age	F%	Dose	Route of Administration	Lumbar Spine BMD (% change)	Femoral Neck BMD (% change)	Total Hip BMD (% change)	Fractures/ Comments
Pamidronate[81] (Fan, 2000)	12 mo	53 (23–66)	0	0.5 mg/kg at baseline and 1 mo	IV	NS (vs −6.4)	NS (vs −9.0)	NA	NA
Ibandronate[82] (Grotz, 2001)	12 mo	42 ± 10	30.6	1 mg before and 2 mg at mo 0, 3, 6, 9	IV	−0.96	0.4	NA	Vertebral deformities were reduced by 70%
Etidronate[83] (Arlen, 2001)	12 mo	41 ± 13	44	400 mg for 2 wk, every 12 wk	Oral	4.3	NS	NA	NS
Alendronate[84] (Giannini, 2001)	24 mo	57 ± 11	35	10 mg/d (with 0.50 µg/d of oral calcitriol)	Oral	5.0	4.5	3.9	NA
Pamidronate[85] (Coco, 2003)	12 mo	43.8 ± 2.3	61.3	Within 48 h and at mo 1, 2, 3, 6	IV	−0.63 (vs −4.6)	NS	NS	NS
Zoledronate[86] (Haas, 2003)	6 mo	55 ± 18	60	4 mg within 2 wk + at mo 3	IV	3.3	−2.9% (NS)	NA	NA
Calcitriol[87] (Torres, 2004)	12 mo	47 ± 12	17.8	0.5 µg every other day	Oral	−3.88	NS	NS	Less bone loss at femoral neck, similar at spine
Alfacalcidol[88] (in children/ adolescents) (El-Husseini, 2004)	12 mo	14.5 ± 3.8	20	0.25 µg/d	Oral	Significant Improvement in T-score	Significant Improvement in T-score	NA	None

(continued on next page)

Table 6
(continued)

Molecule	Duration	Age	F%	Dose	Route of Administration	Lumbar Spine BMD (% change)	Femoral Neck BMD (% change)	Total Hip BMD (% change)	Fractures/ Comments
Alendronate[89] (Toro, 2005)	411 ± 107 d	59.2 ± 6.6	84	70 mg weekly	Oral	NS	5.57	NA	NA
Risedronate[90] (Torregrosa, 2007)	12 mo	58 ± 9	48.7	35 mg weekly	Oral	Significant Improvement in T-score	NS	NA	Fewer vertebral fractures than control (NS)
Alendronate + Alfacalcidol[91] (Trabulus, 2008)	12 mo	35.2 ± 7.7	23.5	10 mg daily + 0.5 μg daily	Oral	Significant Improvement in T-score	Significant Improvement in T-score	NA	No clinical fractures observed
Pamidronate[92] (Walsh, 2009)	12 mo	46.1 ± 12.8	23.9	1 mg/kg at baseline and mo 1, 4, 8, 12	IV	+2.1 (vs −5.7)	Stable (NS)	Stable (vs −4.4)	3.3% and 6.4%, respectively in treatment and control groups
Denosumab[46] (Bonani, 2016)	12 mo	50 ± 14	23.9	60 mg every 6 mo in first year	SC	4.6	NS	2.3	Only one traumatic rib fracture in the control group (Calcium and Vit. D3); no fractures in the denosumab group
Zoledronate[93] (Marques, 2019)	12 mo	43 ± 11	43.8	5 mg shortly after transplantation	IV	5.6	5.8	12.5	Nonsignificant changes in BMD vs control. None of the patients experienced fractures.

Abbreviations: BMD, bone mineral density; F, female; IV, intravenous; NA, not available; NS, nonsignificant; Vit., vitamin.

Denosumab was safely and effectively administered at baseline and 6 months post-transplant in an open-label randomized prospective study involving 90 patients.[46] The results of the trial demonstrated significant hip and spine BMD gain and a steady reduction in BTMs (ß-CTX, BSAP, and P1NP). A traumatic rib fracture was reported in the control group, with none in the treated group. Denosumab is now under evaluation in two other clinical trials (ClinicalTrials.gov Identifier: NCT04169698 and NCT03960554).

Hematopoietic Stem-Cell, Lung, and Small Intestinal Transplantation

Patients undergoing hematopoietic SCT sustain significant bone loss in the first 12 months, especially at the femoral neck. Allogeneic transplantation is characterized by greater bone loss compared with autologous SCT.[47] This may be due to a higher frequency of graft-versus-host disease in the former, leading to intestinal malabsorption or longer exposure to corticosteroid therapy. Fracture rates are nine times higher than in age- and sex-matched controls.[48] Besides high-dose glucocorticoids, prior chemotherapy, total body irradiation and hypogonadism are the main contributory factors to bone loss in SCT-induced osteoporosis. Bisphosphonates and hormone replacement therapy in women have shown efficacy in reducing BMD loss. Denosumab may be a promising agent in SCT due to its significant effect on cortical bone and lack of renal toxicity compared with bisphosphonates.[49] A clinical trial is currently evaluating denosumab in allogenic SCT in the first year posttransplant (ClinicalTrials.gov Identifier: NCT03925532).

Osteoporosis is a common comorbidity in lung transplant recipients. These patients often have had long-term glucocorticoid exposure due to their underlying lung disease, and frequently have lower BMD at transplantation than other transplant groups. Prevalence of osteoporosis may be as high as 73% in patients undergoing lung transplantation, with rates of bone loss and fractures greatest in the first year after transplantation.[30] Increased cortical porosity, trabecular thinning and dropout, and resultant decreased biomechanical properties have recently been documented.[50] Patients with cystic fibrosis may be at even higher risk of osteoporosis because of concomitant pancreatic insufficiency and, consequently, calcium and vitamin D malabsorption. Few osteoporosis medications have been tested in lung transplantation recipients.

Little information is available regarding Small Bowel Transplantation (SBT)-induced osteoporosis. In the largest available retrospective study evaluating 16 patients before and after intestinal transplantation,[36] prevalence of osteoporosis was 6% before transplantation and increased up to 38% over the first year posttransplant. The greatest bone loss was observed at the femoral neck and total hip, with 15% mean loss at both sites. Calcium and vitamin D alone were not able to prevent bone loss at the femoral site. Alendronate significantly reduced BMD loss both at total hip and femoral neck, whereas lumbar spine BMD was unchanged with or without antiresorptive therapy. In this population, prompt administration of intravenous bisphosphonates or denosumab before or after transplantation might be beneficial, with correction of potential risk factors for hypocalcemia.

SUMMARY

Although much is known about the pathophysiology of bone loss and fractures in GIOP and transplant-induced osteoporosis, these conditions remain widely under-treated. Further therapeutic options may be available within several years for transplant recipients after completion of current randomized controlled trials. The natural history of fractures in transplant patients is poorly studied, but fractures appear to increase shortly after transplantation, and then to stabilize at lower rates over the long-term. Anabolic therapies may be useful in transplant-related bone disease if they are able to stimulate reduced bone formation due to glucocorticoid therapy or late-stage chronic kidney disease.

CLINICS CARE POINTS

- Calcium and vitamin D supplementation is necessary but not sufficient to prevent bone loss and fractures in both GIOP and transplant-induced osteoporosis.
- Bisphosphonates are the first-line treatment in GIOP and transplantation osteoporosis, but teriparatide may be more effective due to its anabolic effects in those without contraindications.
- Anabolic therapy with teriparatide is very effective in GIOP, and may be effective in transplant-related osteoporosis as long as patients do not have preexisting hyperparathyroidism.
- Denosumab has shown favorable effects on hip and spine BMD in GIOP and renal transplant patients, with data on fractures lacking.

DISCLOSURE

The authors have nothing to disclose.

REFERENCES

1. Chiodini I, Merlotti D, Falchetti A, et al. Treatment options for glucocorticoid-induced osteoporosis. Expert Opin Pharmacother 2020;21(6):721–32.
2. Cooper MS, Rabbitt EH, Goddard PE, et al. Osteoblastic 11 β-hydroxysteroid dehydrogenase type 1 activity increases with age and glucocorticoid exposure. J Bone Miner Res 2002;17(6):979–86.
3. Weinstein RS. Glucocorticoid-induced osteoporosis and osteonecrosis. Endocrinol Metab Clin North Am 2012;41(3):595–611.
4. Steinbuch M, Youket TE, Cohen S. Oral glucocorticoid use is associated with an increased risk of fracture. Osteoporos Int 2004;15(4):323–8.
5. Kimberg DV, Baerg RD, Gershon E, et al. Effect of cortisone treatment on the active transport of calcium by the small intestine. J Clin Invest 1971;50(6):1309–21.
6. Favus MJ, Kimberg DV, Millar GN, et al. Effects of cortisone administration on the metabolism and localization of 25-hydroxycholecalciferol in the rat. J Clin Invest 1973;52(6):1328–35.
7. Suzuki Y, Ichikawa Y, Saito E, et al. Importance of increased urinary calcium excretion in the development of secondary hyperparathyroidism of patients under glucocorticoid therapy. Metabolism 1983;32(2):151–6.
8. Turner ST, Kiebzak GM, Dousa TP. Mechanism of glucocorticoid effect on renal transport of phosphate. Am J Physiol 1982;243(5):C227–36.
9. Mazziotti G, Formenti AM, Adler RA, et al. Glucocorticoid-induced osteoporosis: pathophysiological role of GH/IGF-I and PTH/Vitamin D axes, treatment options and guidelines. Endocrine 2016;54(3):603–11.
10. Weinstein RS, Wan C, Liu Q, et al. Endogenous glucocorticoids decrease skeletal angiogenesis, vascularity, hydration, and strength in aged mice. Aging Cell 2010;9(2):147–61.

11. Minetto MA, D'Angelo V, Arvat E, et al. Diagnostic work-up in steroid myopathy. Endocrine 2018;60(2):219–23.

12. Humphrey EL, Williams JHH, Davie MWJ, et al. Effects of dissociated glucocorticoids on OPG and RANKL in osteoblastic cells. Bone 2006;38(5):652–61.

13. Chotiyarnwong P, McCloskey EV. Pathogenesis of glucocorticoid-induced osteoporosis and options for treatment. Nat Rev Endocrinol 2020;16(8):437–47.

14. Schepper JD, Collins F, Rios-Arce ND, et al. Involvement of the gut microbiota and barrier function in glucocorticoid-induced osteoporosis. J Bone Miner Res 2019;35(4):801–20.

15. Martineau P, Leslie WD, Johansson H, et al. In which patients does lumbar spine trabecular bone score (TBS) have the largest effect? Bone 2018;113:161–8.

16. Graeff C, Marin F, Petto H, et al. High resolution quantitative computed tomography-based assessment of trabecular microstructure and strength estimates by finite-element analysis of the spine, but not DXA, reflects vertebral fracture status in men with glucocorticoid-induced osteoporosis. Bone 2013;52(2):568–77.

17. Van Staa TP, Leufkens HGM, Abenhaim L, et al. Oral corticosteroids and fracture risk: relationship to daily and cumulative doses. Rheumatology 2000;39(12):1383–9.

18. Buckley L, Humphrey MB. Glucocorticoid-induced osteoporosis. N Engl J Med 2018;379(26):2547–56.

19. Van Staa TP, Leufkens HGM, Abenhaim L, et al. Use of oral corticosteroids and risk of fractures. J Bone Miner Res 2000;15(6):993–1000.

20. Li D, Jeet Kaur R, Ladefoged Ebbehøj A, et al. *Abstract:* MON-219 Prevalence and incidence of fractures in patients with adrenal adenomas: a population-based study of 1003 patients. J Endocr Soc 2020;4(Supplement_1). MON–219.

21. De Vries F, Bracke M, Leufkens HGM, et al. Fracture risk with intermittent high-dose oral glucocorticoid therapy. Arthritis Rheum 2007;56(1):208–14.

22. Kanis JA, Johansson H, Oden A, et al. Guidance for the adjustment of FRAX according to the dose of glucocorticoids. Osteoporos Int 2011;22(3):809–16.

23. Belaya ZE, Iljin AV, Melnichenko GA, et al. Diagnostic performance of osteocalcin measurements in patients with endogenous Cushing's syndrome. Bonekey Rep 2016;5:815.

24. Athimulam S, Delivanis D, Thomas M, et al. The impact of mild autonomous cortisol secretion on bone turnover markers. J Clin Endocrinol Metab 2020;105(5):1469–77.

25. Chandler H, Brooks DJ, Hattersley G, et al. Abaloparatide increases bone mineral density and bone strength in ovariectomized rabbits with glucocorticoid-induced osteopenia. Osteoporos Int 2019;30(8):1607–16.

26. Lan G, Xie X, Peng L, et al. Current status of research on osteoporosis after solid organ transplantation: pathogenesis and management. Biomed Res Int 2015;2015:413169.

27. Campistol JM, Holt DW, Epstein S, et al. Bone metabolism in renal transplant patients treated with cyclosporine or sirolimus. Transpl Int 2005;18(9):1028–35.

28. Singha UK, Jiang Y, Yu S, et al. Rapamycin inhibits osteoblast proliferation and differentiation in MC3T3-E1 cells and primary mouse bone marrow stromal cells. J Cell Biochem 2008;103(2):434–46.

29. Chen J, Long F. MTOR signaling in skeletal development and disease. Bone Res 2018;6(1):1.

30. Ebeling PR. Transplantation osteoporosis. In: Bilezikian JP, editor. Primer on the Metabolic Bone Diseases and Disorders of Mineral Metabolism, ed. 9. Hoboken (NJ): Wiley; 2018. p. 424-31.

31. Majumdar SR, Ezekowitz JA, Lix LM, et al. Heart failure is a clinically and densito-metrically independent risk factor for osteoporotic fractures: population-based cohort study of 45,509 subjects. J Clin Endocrinol Metab 2012;97(4):1179–86.

32. Monegal A, Navasa M, Guañabens N, et al. Bone disease after liver transplanta-tion: a long-term prospective study of bone mass changes, hormonal status and histomorphometric characteristics. Osteoporos Int 2001;12(6):484–92.

33. Alem AM, Sherrard DJ, Gillen DL, et al. Increased risk of hip fracture among pa-tients with end-stage renal disease. Kidney Int 2000;58(1):396–9.

34. Schulte C, Beelen DW, Schaefer UW, et al. Bone loss in long-term survivors after transplantation of hematopoietic stem cells: a prospective study. Osteoporos Int 2000;11(4):344–53.

35. Tschopp O, Boehler A, Speich R, et al. Osteoporosis before lung transplantation: association with low body mass index, but not with underlying disease. Am J Transplant 2002;2(2):167–72.

36. Resnick J, Gupta N, Wagner J, et al. Skeletal integrity and visceral transplanta-tion. Am J Transplant 2010;10(10):2331–40.

37. Seguro LFBC, Pereira RMR, Seguro LPC, et al. Bone metabolism impairment in heart transplant: results from a prospective cohort study. Transplantation 2020; 104(4):873–80.

38. Kerschan-Schindl K, Ruzicka M, Mahr S, et al. Unexpected low incidence of vertebral fractures in heart transplant recipients: analysis of bone turnover. Transpl Int 2008;21(3):255–62.

39. Löfdahl E, Söderlund C, Rådegran G. Bone mineral density and osteoporosis in heart transplanted patients: a single-center retrospective study at Skåne Univer-sity Hospital in Lund 1988-2016. Clin Transplant 2019;33(3):1–9.

40. Leidig-Bruckner G, Hosch S, Dodidou P, et al. Frequency and predictors of oste-oporotic fractures after cardiac or liver transplantation: a follow-up study. Lancet 2001;357(9253):342–7.

41. Guichelaar MM, Malinchoc M, Sibonga JD, et al. Bone histomorphometric changes after liver transplantation for chronic cholestatic liver disease. J Bone Miner Res 2003;18(12):2190–9.

42. de Kroon L, Drent G, van den Berg AP, et al. Liver Transplant Group Groningen. Current health status of patients who have survived for more than 15 years after liver transplantation. Neth J Med 2007;65(7):252–8.

43. Kasturi KS, Chennareddygari S, Mummadi RR. Effect of bisphosphonates on bone mineral density in liver transplant patients: a meta-analysis and systematic review of randomized controlled trials. Transpl Int 2010;23(2):200–7.

44. Brunova J, Kratochvilova S, Stepankova J. Osteoporosis therapy with denosu-mab in organ transplant recipients. Front Endocrinol (Lausanne) 2018;9:1–8.

45. Julian BA, Laskow DA, Dubovsky J, et al. Rapid loss of vertebral mineral density after renal transplantation. N Engl J Med 1991;325(8):544–50.

46. Bonani M, Frey D, Brockmann J, et al. Effect of twice-yearly denosumab on pre-vention of bone mineral density loss in de novo kidney transplant recipients: a randomized controlled trial. Am J Transplant 2016;16(6):1882–91.

47. Ebeling PR, Thomas DM, Erbas B, et al. Mechanisms of bone loss following allo-geneic and autologous hemopoietic stem cell transplantation. J Bone Miner Res 1999;14(3):342–50.

48. Pundole XN, Barbo AG, Lin H, et al. Increased incidence of fractures in recipients of hematopoietic stem-cell transplantation. J Clin Oncol 2015;33(12):1364–70.

49. Kendler DL, Body JJ, Brandi ML, et al. Bone management in hematologic stem cell transplant recipients. Osteoporos Int 2018;29(12):2597–610.

50. Fischer L, Valentinitsch A, DiFranco MD, et al. High-resolution peripheral quantitative CT imaging: cortical porosity, poor trabecular bone microarchitecture, and low bone strength in lung transplant recipients. Radiology 2015;274(2):473–81.

51. Saag KG, Emkey R, Schnitzer TJ, et al. Alendronate for the prevention and treatment of glucocorticoid-induced osteoporosis. N Engl J Med 1998;339(5):292–9.

52. Wallach S, Cohen S, Reid DM, et al. Effects of risedronate treatment on bone density and vertebral fracture in patients on corticosteroid therapy. Calcif Tissue Int 2000;67(4):277–85.

53. Adachi JD, Saag KG, Delmas PD, et al. Two-year effects of alendronate on bone mineral density and vertebral fracture in patients receiving glucocorticoids: A randomized, double-blind, placebo-controlled extension trial. Arthritis Rheum 2001;44(1):202–11.

54. de Nijs RNJ, Jacobs JWG, Lems WF, et al. Alendronate or alfacalcidol in glucocorticoid-induced osteoporosis. N Engl J Med 2006;355(7):675–84.

55. Saag KG, Shane E, Boonen S, et al. Teriparatide or alendronate in glucocorticoid-induced osteoporosis. N Engl J Med 2007;357(20):2028–39.

56. Saag KG, Zanchetta JR, Devogelaer JP, et al. Effects of teriparatide versus alendronate for treating glucocorticoid-induced osteoporosis: Thirty-six-month results of a randomized, double-blind, controlled trial. Arthritis Rheum 2009; 60(11):3346–55.

57. Stoch SA, Saag KG, Greenwald M, et al. Once-weekly oral alendronate 70 mg in patients with glucocorticoid-induced bone loss: A 12-month randomized, placebo-controlled clinical trial. J Rheumatol 2009;36(8):1705–14.

58. Mok CC, Ying KY, To CH, et al. Raloxifene for prevention of glucocorticoid-induced bone loss: a 12-month randomised double-blinded placebo-controlled trial. Ann Rheum Dis 2011;70(5):778–84.

59. Hakala M, Kröger H, Valleala H, et al. Once-monthly oral ibandronate provides significant improvement in bone mineral density in postmenopausal women treated with glucocorticoids for inflammatory rheumatic diseases: A 12-month, randomized, double-blind, placebo-controlled trial. Scand J Rheumatol 2012; 41(4):260–6.

60. Sambrook PN, Roux C, Devogelaer JP, et al. Bisphosphonates and glucocorticoid osteoporosis in men: Results of a randomized controlled trial comparing zoledronic acid with risedronate. Bone 2012;50(1):289–95.

61. Glüer CC, Marin F, Ringe JD, et al. Comparative effects of teriparatide and risedronate in glucocorticoid-induced osteoporosis in men: 18-month results of the EuroGIOPs trial. J Bone Miner Res 2013;28(6):1355–68.

62. Saag KG, Wagman RB, Geusens P, et al. Denosumab versus risedronate in glucocorticoid-induced osteoporosis: a multicentre, randomised, double-blind, active-controlled, double-dummy, non-inferiority study. Lancet Diabetes Endocrinol 2018;6(6):445–54.

63. Saag KG, Pannacciulli N, Geusens P, et al. Denosumab versus risedronate in glucocorticoid-induced osteoporosis: final results of a twenty-four–month randomized, double-blind, double-dummy trial. Arthritis Rheumatol 2019;71(7): 1174–84.

64. Garcia-Delgado I, Prieto S, Gil-Fraguas L, et al. Calcitonin, etidronate, and calcidiol treatment in bone loss after cardiac transplantation. Calcif Tissue Int 1997; 60(2):155–9.
65. Shane E, Rodino MA, McMahon DJ, et al. Prevention of bone loss after heart transplantation with antiresorptive therapy: a pilot study. J Heart Lung Transplant 1998;17(11):1089–96.
66. Sambrook P, Henderson NK, Keogh A, et al. Effect of calcitriol on bone loss after cardiac or lung transplantation. J Bone Miner Res 2000;15(9):1818–24.
67. Bianda T, Linka A, Junga G, et al. Prevention of osteoporosis in heart transplant recipients: A comparison of calcitriol with calcitonin and pamidronate. Calcif Tissue Int 2000;67(2):116–21.
68. Krieg MA, Seydoux C, Sandini L, et al. Intravenous pamidronate as treatment for osteoporosis after heart transplantation: a prospective study. Osteoporos Int 2001;12(2):112–6.
69. Ippoliti G, Pellegrini C, Campana C, et al. Clodronate treatment of established bone loss in cardiac recipients: a randomized study. Transplantation 2003; 75(3):330–4.
70. Shane E, Addesso V, Namerow PB, et al. Alendronate versus calcitriol for the prevention of bone loss after cardiac transplantation. N Engl J Med 2004;350(8): 767–76.
71. Fahrleitner-Pammer A, Piswanger-Soelkner JC, Pieber TR, et al. Ibandronate prevents bone loss and reduces vertebral fracture risk in male cardiac transplant patients: a randomized double-blind, placebo-controlled trial. J Bone Miner Res 2009;24(7):1335–44.
72. Lange U, Classen K, Müller-Ladner U, et al. Weekly oral bisphosphonates over 2 years prevent bone loss in cardiac transplant patients. Clin Transplant 2017; 31(11):e13122.
73. Crawford BAL, Kam C, Pavlovic J, et al. Zoledronic acid prevents bone loss after liver transplantation: a randomized, double-blind, placebo-controlled trial. Ann Intern Med 2006;144(4):239–48.
74. Pennisi P, Trombetti A, Giostra E, et al. Pamidronate and osteoporosis prevention in liver transplant recipients. Rheumatol Int 2006;27(3):251–6.
75. Atamaz F, Hepguler S, Karasu Z, et al. The prevention of bone fractures after liver transplantation: experience with alendronate treatment. Transplant Proc 2006; 38(5):1448–52.
76. Bodingbauer M, Wekerle T, Pakrah B, et al. Prophylactic bisphosphonate treatment prevents bone fractures after liver transplantation. Am J Transplant 2007; 7(7):1763–9.
77. Monegal A, Guañabens N, Suárez MJ, et al. Pamidronate in the prevention of bone loss after liver transplantation: a randomized controlled trial. Transpl Int 2009;22(2):198–206.
78. Kaemmerer D, Lehmann G, Wolf G, et al. Treatment of osteoporosis after liver transplantation with ibandronate. Transpl Int 2010;23(7):753–9.
79. Guadalix S, Martínez-Díaz-Guerra G, Lora D, et al. Effect of early risedronate treatment on bone mineral density and bone turnover markers after liver transplantation: a prospective single-center study. Transpl Int 2011;24(7):657–65.
80. Shane E, Cohen A, Stein EM, et al. Zoledronic acid versus alendronate for the prevention of bone loss after heart or liver transplantation. J Clin Endocrinol Metab 2012;97(12):4481–90.
81. Fan SLS, Almond MK, Ball E, et al. Pamidronate therapy as prevention of bone loss following renal transplantation. Kidney Int 2000;57(2):684–90.

82. Grotz W, Nagel C, Poeschel D, et al. Effect of ibandronate on bone loss and renal function after kidney transplantation. J Am Soc Nephrol 2001;12(7):1530–7.

83. Arlen DJ, Lambert K, Ioannidis G, et al. Treatment of established bone loss after renal transplantation with etidronate. Transplantation 2001;71(5):669–73.

84. Giannini S, D'Angelo A, Carraro G, et al. Alendronate prevents further bone loss in renal transplant recipients. J Bone Miner Res 2001;16(11):2111–7.

85. Coco M, Glicklich D, Faugere MC, et al. Prevention of bone loss in renal transplant recipients: A prospective, randomized trial of intravenous pamidronate. J Am Soc Nephrol 2003;14(10):2669–76.

86. Haas M, Leko-Mohr Z, Roschger P, et al. Zoledronic acid to prevent bone loss in the first 6 months after renal transplantation. Kidney Int 2003;63(3):1130–6.

87. Torres A, García S, Gómez A, et al. Treatment with intermittent calcitriol and calcium reduces bone loss after renal transplantation. Kidney Int 2004;65(2):705–12.

88. El-Husseini AA, El-Agroudy AE, El-Sayed M, et al. A prospective randomized study for the treatment of bone loss with vitamin D during kidney transplantation in children and adolescents. Am J Transplant 2004;4(12):2052–7.

89. Toro J, Gentil MA, García R, et al. Alendronate in kidney transplant patients: a single-center experience. Transplant Proc 2005;37(3):1471–2.

90. Torregrosa JV, Fuster D, Pedroso S, et al. Weekly risedronate in kidney transplant patients with osteopenia. Transpl Int 2007;20(8):708–11.

91. Trabulus S, Altiparmak MR, Apaydin S, et al. Treatment of renal transplant recipients with low bone mineral density: a randomized prospective trial of alendronate, alfacalcidol, and alendronate combined with alfacalcidol. Transplant Proc 2008;40(1):160–6.

92. Walsh SB, Altmann P, Pattison J, et al. Effect of pamidronate on bone loss after kidney transplantation: a randomized trial. Am J Kidney Dis 2009;53(5):856–65.

93. Marques IDB, Araújo MJCLN, Graciolli FG, et al. A randomized trial of zoledronic acid to prevent bone loss in the first year after kidney transplantation. J Am Soc Nephrol 2019;30(2):355–65.

Diabetes and Osteoporosis
Part I, Epidemiology and Pathophysiology

G. Isanne Schacter, MD, FRCPC[a], William D. Leslie, MD, FRCPC, MSc[b],*

KEYWORDS

- Diabetes • Bone • Osteoporosis • Fracture • Bone mineral density
- Dual-energy x-ray absorptiometry

KEY POINTS

- Both Type 1 and 2 diabetes mellitus are associated with an increased risk of fracture.
- The pathogenesis of diabetes-induced osteoporosis differs between Type 1 and 2 diabetes mellitus.
- Some antidiabetic medications, especially thiazolidinediones, may contribute to increased risk of fracture in diabetes.

BACKGROUND

Both diabetes and osteoporosis are increasingly prevalent diseases, in part owing to aging populations.[1,2] According to the World Health Organization, diabetes mellitus is present in more than 463 million individuals worldwide, with numbers expected to double by 2040.[1] Type 1 diabetes (T1D) is present in fewer than 10% of adults with diabetes, but the prevalence is increasing by 2% to 3% per year.[3] Type 2 diabetes (T2D) currently affects almost 22% of older adults in the United States (including diagnosed and undiagnosed cases).[4]

Epidemiologic data have shown that other organs may be adversely affected by diabetes, including the skeleton, in what has become known as diabetes-induced osteoporosis. Diabetes-induced osteoporosis represents the combined impact of conventional osteoporosis with the additional fracture burden attributed to diabetes. A conceptual framework for this increase in fracture burden is illustrated in **Fig. 1**.

The authors have nothing to disclose.
[a] Department of Medicine, Rady Faculty of Health Sciences, University of Manitoba, GF-335, 820 Sherbrook Street, Winnipeg, Manitoba R3A 1R9, Canada; [b] Department of Medicine, Rady Faculty of Health Sciences, University of Manitoba, C5121, 409 Tache Avenue, Winnipeg, Manitoba R2H 2A6, Canada
* Corresponding author.
E-mail address: bleslie@sbgh.mb.ca

Endocrinol Metab Clin N Am 50 (2021) 275–285
https://doi.org/10.1016/j.ecl.2021.03.005
0889-8529/21/© 2021 Elsevier Inc. All rights reserved.

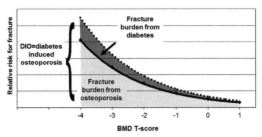

Fig. 1. Conceptual framework for diabetes and fractures. The light gray region below the solid line indicates the fracture burden attributable to osteoporosis; the dark gray region between the dotted and solid lines indicates the additional fracture burden attributable to diabetes. (*From* Schacter GI, Leslie WD. DXA-Based Measurements in Diabetes: Can They Predict Fracture Risk? Calcif Tissue Int 2017;100:150-164; with permission.)

EPIDEMIOLOGY
Fracture Incidence

Many studies have confirmed an increased risk of fracture in patients with T1D and T2D, but this is much greater in the former and cannot be explained from reductions in bone mineral density (BMD).[5–8] The most recent meta-analysis from Vilaca and colleagues[9] (47 included studies up to March 2020) reported a relative risk (RR) for hip fracture of RR 4.93 (95% confidence interval [CI] 3.06-7.95) in T1D and RR 1.33 (95% CI 1.19–1.49) in T2D. Hip fracture risk was even higher in those younger than 65 years for both T1D and T2D. In T2D, the risk of hip fractures was higher in women, insulin users, and those with disease duration of more than 10 years. Nonvertebral fractures were also increased in T1D (RR 1.92, 95% CI 0.92–3.99) and T2D (RR 1.19, 95% CI 1.11–1.28).

A meta-analysis from Wang and colleagues[10] reported detailed site-specific fracture outcomes. Diabetes overall (T1D and T2D combined) was associated with an increased risk of total (RR 1.32%, 95% CI 1.17–1.48), hip (RR 1.77%, 95% CI 1.56–2.02), upper arm (RR 1.47%, 95% CI 1.02–2.10), and ankle fractures (RR 1.24%, 95% CI 1.10–1.40), but not on distal forearm fractures (RR 1.02%, 95% CI 0.88–1.19). There was a nonsignificant trend to greater risk for vertebral fractures (RR 1.56%, 95% CI 0.78–3.12). Patients with T1D had greater risk of total ($P = .002$), hip ($P < .001$), and ankle fractures ($P = .029$) as compared with those with T2D.

Koromani and colleagues[11] analyzed data from 15 studies comprising more than 850,000 subjects, and found that individuals with T2D had increased vertebral fracture risk (odds ratio [OR] 1.35, 95% CI 1.27–1.44). Individual participant data cohorts (N = 19,820) revealed that the risk of incident nonvertebral fractures was higher in those with both T2D and prior vertebral fracture compared with those without either (hazard ratio [HR] 2.42, 95% CI 1.86–3.15), those with prior vertebral fracture alone (HR 1.73, 95% CI 1.32–2.27), and T2D alone (HR 1.94, 95% CI 1.46–2.59). Individuals with both T2D and vertebral fracture had increased mortality compared with individuals without either (HR 2.11, 95% CI 1.72–2.59), those with vertebral fractures alone (HR 1.84, 95% CI 1.49–2.28), and those with T2D alone (HR 1.23, 95% CI 0.99–1.52).

RISK FACTORS FOR FRACTURE
Type 1 Diabetes

There has been a long-established association between T1D and osteoporosis.[6] The increase in fracture risk (particularly marked at the hip) is much greater than expected on the basis of the BMD decrement, implying that there are other BMD-independent factors that contribute to this increased fracture risk.[12,13]

Risk factors associated with lower BMD in T1D include male gender,[14,15] longer duration of disease,[16] younger age at diagnosis,[17] lower endogenous insulin and/or C-peptide levels,[18] lower body mass index (BMI),[19] and potentially the comorbidities and/or chronic autoimmunity associated with a chronic disease.[20] Other reported factors include the presence of microvascular complications[21] (retinopathy,[22] neuropathy,[23] and nephropathy).[24] Risk factors for fracture in T1D include the presence of T1D itself,[5] longer duration of disease,[5] female sex,[5,9] microvascular complications,[25] long-term glycemic control, and decreased vitamin D levels.[26] This risk is amplified by the increase in risk of falls, which can be a consequence of hypoglycemia, visual defects, peripheral neuropathy, or other disability.[27]

Type 2 Diabetes

T2D and low-trauma fracture both become more common with advancing age. T2D is associated with both greater weight and higher BMD.[28] Although both were historically assumed to be protective against fracture, a paradoxic increased risk of fracture has been observed in T2D as noted earlier, though this risk is generally smaller than in T1D. In the Health, Aging and Body Composition study, Strotmeyer and colleagues[29] found that T2D was associated with higher hip, whole body, and volumetric spine BMD, which was independent of body composition and fasting insulin levels. The same cohort noted increased fracture risk in those with diabetes even after adjustment for age, calcaneal BMD, BMI, and other covariates.[30]

Risk factors for fracture in T2D include older age,[31] lower BMD, lower BMI, and falls.[32] Similar to T1D, diabetes duration,[9,31] and diabetes complications[25] are both associated with increased risk. The diabetes-fracture association may also differ between populations. In data from the National Health and Nutrition Examination Survey, Looker and colleagues[33] found the association between fracture risk and diabetes to differ significantly by race/ethnicity (P for interaction $<.05$).

PATHOPHYSIOLOGY

The pathophysiology of increased fracture risk in T1D and T2D differs, although both involve relatively reduced bone formation, osteoblast dysfunction, and low bone turnover. Starup-Linde and colleagues[34] demonstrated in a meta-analysis of 22 studies that when comparing biochemical bone turnover among patients with diabetes and controls, significant (although modest) reductions were seen among patients with diabetes for osteocalcin (-1.15 ng/mL [range, -1.78 to -0.52]) and C-terminal cross-linked telopeptide (-0.14 ng/mL [range, -0.22 to -0.05]). T1D is associated with decreased BMD, whereas in T2D, BMD is frequently increased or normal,[35–37] implying that the pathophysiology of diabetes-induced osteoporosis is multifactorial. To date, there have been an insufficient number of studies stratified according to diabetes type to directly compare T1D and T2D.

Diabetes and hyperglycemia are associated with hyperlipidemia, decreased insulin signaling, decreased insulinlike growth factor 1 (IGF-1), reactive oxygen species production,[38] and inflammation, all of which could potentially contribute to suppression of osteoblast activity. Both obesity and diabetes itself can increase bone marrow inflammation, resulting in the impairment of osteoblast activity.[39] The inflammation favors an increase in osteoclast number and activity, leading to increased bone loss.[40] In both T1D[41] and T2D,[42] increased levels of inflammatory cytokines have been demonstrated. Multiple factors could potentially contribute to degraded bone quality and microarchitectural defects,[28] including chronic hyperglycemia,[37] and skeletal advanced glycation end products (AGES),[43] which irreversibly accrue from the nonenzymatic addition of sugar moieties to the amine groups of proteins,[44,45] and then have a subsequent negative impact on skeletal integrity,[46] particularly type 1 collagen. Oxidative stress is increased by hyperglycemia via 2 mechanisms: (1) glucose overloads the mitochondria, and (2) AGEs and polyol signaling.[47] This oxidative stress in turn negatively affects osteoblast maturation,[48] and may also trigger an increase in osteoblast apoptosis.[49] AGEs increase collagen cross-linking, which causes change to the structural and functional properties of proteins (contributing to overall decreased bone strength and increased brittleness), and their levels correlate with the severity of diabetes complications.[50] Due to low bone turnover, there is greater opportunity for proteins to accumulate AGEs, and so these levels are especially high in patients with diabetes.[51] Chronically increased glucose levels promote bone matrix glycation, while impairing collagen turnover and matrix renewal, leading to the end result of impaired bone formation and more fragile bones containing higher levels of AGEs per gram of collagen. These collagen modifications stiffen the bone matrix and modify bone's material properties, leading to brittleness and mechanical failure under physiologic levels of stress.[52,53]

In T1D, several mechanisms have been proposed to account for the skeletal fragility and deficits in BMD, bone geometry, bone microarchitecture, and biomechanical properties.[50,54–57] The primary bone derangement is decreased bone formation secondary to decreased osteoblast activity.[50,58,59] Lower levels of IGF-1 and procollagen type 1 amino-terminal propeptide (P1NP) in individuals with T1D may also play a prominent role.[50,60] The detrimental effects of AGEs on bone tissue in vivo are reflected by the presence of increased pentosidine, a marker of AGEs, on bone histomorphometry in individuals with T1D with prevalent fractures, compared with those without fracture.[61]

A potential connection between diabetes and serum osteocalcin has been suggested.[62] In patients with either T1D or T2D, serum osteocalcin is lower than in controls without diabetes.[63–65] Moreover, osteocalcin is negatively correlated with glycosylated hemoglobin levels in patients with T1D.[64]

As diabetes is marked by reduced bone turnover and osteoblast activity, a role for altered Wnt signaling has been suggested.[66,67] Sclerostin is an osteocyte product that antagonizes the Wnt signaling pathway, and increased levels inhibit bone formation,[66] with an end result of uncoupling of bone formation and resorption.

ANTIDIABETIC MEDICATIONS

Antidiabetic medications may also contribute to increased risk of fracture in diabetes (**Table 1**). This risk has been most consistently seen in association with thiazolidinedione (TZD), which has been shown to have direct detrimental effects on bone health in humans. In an updated meta-analysis (studies to February 2019) from Hidayat and colleagues,[68] both pioglitazone (RR 1.38, 95% CI 1.23–1.54) and rosiglitazone (RR 1.34, 95% CI 1.14–1.58) were positively associated with the risk of fracture.

Metformin has not been found to consistently affect either bone mass or fracture risk.[69,70] According to in vitro studies, metformin may exert osteogenic effects via the activation of adenosine monophosphate-activated protein kinase, leading to osteoblastic cell differentiation, bone matrix synthesis, and osteoblast proliferation.[71,72] Some meta-analyses have demonstrated a lower risk of fracture with metformin use.[68,73,74] However, a recent large study from South Korea compared more than 64,000 patients with and without metformin use.[75] After propensity score matching,

Table 1		
Predominant effects of diabetes medications on bone mineral density (BMD) and the fracture risk in type 2 diabetes		
Medications	BMD	Risk of Fracture
Thiazolidinediones	↓	↑
Metformin	No change or ↑	No change or ↓
Sulphonylureas	NA	No change or ↓
Incretins		
GLP-1 agonist	No change or ↑	No change or ↓
DPP-4 inhibitor	No change or ↑	No change or ↓
SGLT-2 inhibitors	No change or ↓	No change
Insulin	No change	↑

Abbreviations: ↑, increase; ↓, decrease; DPP4, dipeptidyl peptidase inhibitor 4; GLP, glucagon-like peptide; NA, not available; SGLT2, sodium/glucose cotransporter 2.

metformin use was not associated with a significant risk of hip fracture (HR 1.00; 95% CI 0.86–1.16).

Sulfonylureas may slightly increase risk of fracture. In an updated meta-analysis (11 studies up to February 2019 containing more than 255,000 subjects), Zhang and colleagues[76] demonstrated that the pooled RR for fracture was increased at 1.14 (95% CI 1.08–1.19) for subjects treated with versus without sulfonylureas, similar to the risk with TZD use, higher than with metformin, but lower than with insulin. Hidayat and colleagues,[68] reported an even higher risk from sulfonylureas (RR 1.30, 95% CI 1.18–1.43). The mechanism underlying this increased risk is unclear but may reflect the increased risk of hypoglycemia and subsequent falls.

Dipeptidyl peptidase-4 (DPP-4) inhibitors and glucagonlike peptide-1 (GLP-1) analogues may have a beneficial effect on bone, possibly through increased levels of serum GLP-1.[77,78] A 2011 meta-analysis (28 trials, 63 fractures) found DPP-4 inhibitors compared with placebo or other treatments were associated with a reduced risk of fracture (OR 0.60, 95% CI 0.37–0.99), even after the exclusion of comparisons with TZDs or sulfonylureas.[79] Cheng and colleagues[80] demonstrated in a recent meta-analysis that use of specific GLP-1 analogues (liraglutide and lixisenatide) were associated with a significant reduction in the risk of fractures (OR 0.71, 95% CI 0.56–0.91), but only with use extended past 52 weeks duration. However, the subsequent meta-analysis from Hidayat and colleagues,[81] did not support an association between the use of DPP-4 inhibitors or GLP-1 analogues and risk of fracture.

Sodium-glucose cotransporter 2 (SGLT-2) inhibitors have attracted much attention recently. A decrease in total hip BMD of up to 1.2% after 2 years of use has been reported, although no changes at other sites were found.[82] In the CANagliflozin cardiovascular Assessment Study (CANVAS), canagliflozin was associated with a higher incidence of fracture primarily affecting the distal extremities within just 12 weeks of initiation of therapy versus placebo (4.0% 2.6%), though inexplicably no excess risk was seen in the parallel renal trial (CANVAS-R).[83,84] These effects may have been related to the osmotic diuresis, volume depletion and weight loss that often accompanies the use of these agents. However, no increased risk was found with canagliflozin in a pooled group of studies outside the CANVAS study.[83] Ruanpeng and colleagues[85] demonstrated a pooled RR of 0.67 (95% CI 0.42–1.07), whereas more recently Azharuddin and colleagues[86] reported in a meta-analysis of more than 32,000 patients with 466 incident fractures that SGLT2 inhibitors were not associated with an increased risk of fracture (OR 1.01, 95% CI 0.83–1.23; P = .91). Fralick and colleagues[87] analyzed 2 US commercial health care databases providing data on more than 70 million patients, with 79,964 patients initiating canagliflozin matched to 79,964 patients initiating a GLP-1 agonist. The primary fracture outcome was similar for canagliflozin and GLP-1 agonists (overall HR 0.98, 95% CI 0.75–1.26) and for the secondary outcome of pelvic, hip, humerus, radius, ulna, carpal, metacarpal, metatarsal, or ankle fracture (HR 0.92, CI 0.83–1.02). Similar results were seen from a nationwide register-based cohort study in Sweden and Denmark of SGLT-2 inhibitors versus GLP-1 receptor agonists (HR 1.11, 95% CI 0.93–1.33).[88] The preponderance of the evidence and most recent meta-analysis suggest that SGLT-2 inhibitors including canagliflozin and GLP-1 agonists are not associated with increased risk for fracture.[81]

Insulin use has been implicated as a possible risk for fracture, but this is confounded by its association with both the longer duration and severity of diabetes itself.[89,90] There have been no randomized trials of insulin therapy with fracture or BMD outcomes. There may be a lower risk for fracture with glargine use as compared with neutral protamine Hagedorn (NPH) insulin.[91] Some studies have reported an increased risk of fracture,[9,31,68,92,93] which has often been attributed to the increased risk of hypoglycemia, and subsequent falls.[76,92,94] Zhang and colleagues[92] examined a total of 7 studies comprising 138,690 patients, and found that insulin was associated with a significantly increased risk of fracture among patients with T2D, when compared with oral antihyperglycemic agents (RR 1.24, 95% CI 1.07–1.44). Subgroup analysis by fracture site indicated that the RR for hip was 1.18 (95% CI 0.83–1.68; P = .363), that for vertebral fracture was 1.28 (95% CI 0.90–1.81) and that for nonvertebral sites was 1.06 (95% CI 0.80–1.41).

SUMMARY

Diabetes-induced osteoporosis in both T1D and T2D is characterized by an increase in fracture risk. As the prevalence of diabetes (especially T2D) continues to increase, increased skeletal complications may follow, and might be exacerbated by some medications used to control hyperglycemia.

CLINICS CARE POINTS

- Both diabetes and osteoporosis are increasingly prevalent diseases, in part owing to aging populations worldwide.
- There is an increased risk of fracture (particularly marked at the hip) in patients with both T1D and T2D, which is much greater than expected based on the BMD decrement implying that there are other BMD-independent factors that contribute to this increased fracture risk.
- Some antidiabetic medications, especially thiazolidinediones, may contribute to increased risk of fracture in diabetes.

REFERENCES

1. IDF diabetes atlas. 2019. Available at: https://diabetesatlas.org/en/. Accessed May 28, 2020].
2. Cole ZA, Dennison EM, Cooper C. Osteoporosis epidemiology update. Curr Rheumatol Rep 2008;10(2):92–6.

3. Atkinson MA, Eisenbarth GS, Michels AW. Type 1 diabetes. Lancet 2014; 383(9911):69–82.
4. Cowie CC, et al. Prevalence of diabetes and impaired fasting glucose in adults in the U.S. population: National Health and Nutrition Examination Survey 1999-2002. Diabetes Care 2006;29(6):1263–8.
5. Formiga F, Freitez Ferreira MD, Montero A. [Diabetes mellitus and risk of hip fracture. A systematic review]. Rev Esp Geriatr Gerontol 2020;55(1):34–41.
6. Shah VN, Shah CS, Snell-Bergeon JK. Type 1 diabetes and risk of fracture: meta-analysis and review of the literature. Diabet Med 2015;32(9):1134–42.
7. Fan Y, et al. Diabetes mellitus and risk of hip fractures: a meta-analysis. Osteoporos Int 2016;27(1):219–28.
8. Janghorbani M, et al. Systematic review of type 1 and type 2 diabetes mellitus and risk of fracture. Am J Epidemiol 2007;166(5):495–505.
9. Vilaca T, et al. The risk of hip and non-vertebral fractures in type 1 and type 2 diabetes: a systematic review and meta-analysis update. Bone 2020;137:115457.
10. Wang H, et al. Diabetes mellitus and the risk of fractures at specific sites: a meta-analysis. BMJ Open 2019;9(1):e024067.
11. Koromani F, et al. Vertebral fractures in individuals with type 2 diabetes: more than skeletal complications alone. Diabetes Care 2020;43(1):137–44.
12. Vestergaard P. Discrepancies in bone mineral density and fracture risk in patients with type 1 and type 2 diabetes–a meta-analysis. Osteoporos Int 2007;18(4): 427–44.
13. Zhukouskaya VV, et al. Prevalence of morphometric vertebral fractures in patients with type 1 diabetes. Diabetes Care 2013;36(6):1635–40.
14. Hamilton EJ, et al. Prevalence and predictors of osteopenia and osteoporosis in adults with Type 1 diabetes. Diabet Med 2009;26(1):45–52.
15. Hamilton EJ, et al. A five-year prospective study of bone mineral density in men and women with diabetes: the Fremantle Diabetes Study. Acta Diabetol 2012; 49(2):153–8.
16. Miazgowski T, Czekalski S. A 2-year follow-up study on bone mineral density and markers of bone turnover in patients with long-standing insulin-dependent diabetes mellitus. Osteoporos Int 1998;8(5):399–403.
17. Maser RE, et al. Hip strength in adults with type 1 diabetes is associated with age at onset of diabetes. J Clin Densitom 2012;15(1):78–85.
18. López-Ibarra PJ, et al. Bone mineral density at time of clinical diagnosis of adult-onset type 1 diabetes mellitus. Endocr Pract 2001;7(5):346–51.
19. Eller-Vainicher C, et al. Low bone mineral density and its predictors in type 1 diabetic patients evaluated by the classic statistics and artificial neural network analysis. Diabetes Care 2011;34(10):2186–91.
20. Lombardi F, et al. Bone involvement in clusters of autoimmune diseases: just a complication? Bone 2010;46(2):551–5.
21. Muñoz-Torres M, et al. Bone mineral density measured by dual X-ray absorptiometry in Spanish patients with insulin-dependent diabetes mellitus. Calcif Tissue Int 1996;58(5):316–9.
22. Campos Pastor MM, et al. Intensive insulin therapy and bone mineral density in type 1 diabetes mellitus: a prospective study. Osteoporos Int 2000;11(5):455–9.
23. Rix M, Andreassen H, Eskildsen P. Impact of peripheral neuropathy on bone density in patients with type 1 diabetes. Diabetes Care 1999;22(5):827–31.
24. Smets YF, et al. Long-term follow-up study on bone mineral density and fractures after simultaneous pancreas-kidney transplantation. Kidney Int 2004;66(5): 2070–6.

25. Vestergaard P, Rejnmark L, Mosekilde L. Diabetes and its complications and their relationship with risk of fractures in type 1 and 2 diabetes. Calcif Tissue Int 2009; 84(1):45–55.

26. Christodoulou S, et al. Vitamin D and bone disease. Biomed Res Int 2013;2013: 396541.

27. Bonds DE, et al. Risk of fracture in women with type 2 diabetes: the Women's Health Initiative Observational Study. J Clin Endocrinol Metab 2006;91(9): 3404–10.

28. Armas LA, et al. Trabecular bone histomorphometry in humans with Type 1 diabetes mellitus. Bone 2012;50(1):91–6.

29. Strotmeyer ES, et al. Diabetes is associated independently of body composition with BMD and bone volume in older white and black men and women: The Health, Aging, and Body Composition Study. J Bone Miner Res 2004;19(7): 1084–91.

30. Schwartz AV, et al. Older women with diabetes have a higher risk of falls: a prospective study. Diabetes Care 2002;25(10):1749–54.

31. Moayeri A, et al. Fracture risk in patients with type 2 diabetes mellitus and possible risk factors: a systematic review and meta-analysis. Ther Clin Risk Manag 2017;13:455–68.

32. Leslie WD, et al. Does diabetes modify the effect of FRAX risk factors for predicting major osteoporotic and hip fracture? Osteoporos Int 2014;25(12):2817–24.

33. Looker AC, Eberhardt MS, Saydah SH. Diabetes and fracture risk in older U.S. adults. Bone 2016;82:9–15.

34. Starup-Linde J, et al. Biochemical markers of bone turnover in diabetes patients–a meta-analysis, and a methodological study on the effects of glucose on bone markers. Osteoporos Int 2014;25(6):1697–708.

35. Oei L, et al. High bone mineral density and fracture risk in type 2 diabetes as skeletal complications of inadequate glucose control: the Rotterdam Study. Diabetes Care 2013;36(6):1619–28.

36. Zhu K, et al. Discordance between fat mass index and body mass index is associated with reduced bone mineral density in women but not in men: the Busselton Healthy Ageing Study. Osteoporos Int 2017;28(1):259–68.

37. Mastrandrea LD, et al. Young women with type 1 diabetes have lower bone mineral density that persists over time. Diabetes Care 2008;31(9):1729–35.

38. McCabe L, Zhang J, Raehtz S. Understanding the skeletal pathology of type 1 and 2 diabetes mellitus. Crit Rev Eukaryot Gene Expr 2011;21(2):187–206.

39. Tsoli M, Boutzios G, Kaltsas G. Immune system effects on the endocrine system. In: Endotext, K.R. Feingold, et al, editors. South Dartmouth, MA: MDText.com, Inc; 2000.

40. Halade GV, et al. Obesity-mediated inflammatory microenvironment stimulates osteoclastogenesis and bone loss in mice. Exp Gerontol 2011;46(1):43–52.

41. Borst SE. The role of TNF-alpha in insulin resistance. Endocrine 2004;23(2–3): 177–82.

42. Katsuki A, et al. Serum levels of tumor necrosis factor-alpha are increased in obese patients with noninsulin-dependent diabetes mellitus. J Clin Endocrinol Metab 1998;83(3):859–62.

43. Yamagishi S. Role of advanced glycation end products (AGEs) in osteoporosis in diabetes. Curr Drug Targets 2011;12(14):2096–102.

44. Ramasamy R, Yan SF, Schmidt AM. The diverse ligand repertoire of the receptor for advanced glycation endproducts and pathways to the complications of diabetes. Vascul Pharmacol 2012;57(5–6):160–7.

45. Tang SY, Vashishth D. The relative contributions of non-enzymatic glycation and cortical porosity on the fracture toughness of aging bone. J Biomech 2011;44(2):330–6.
46. Vashishth D. The role of the collagen matrix in skeletal fragility. Curr Osteoporos Rep 2007;5(2):62–6.
47. Weinberg E, et al. Streptozotocin-induced diabetes in rats diminishes the size of the osteoprogenitor pool in bone marrow. Diabetes Res Clin Pract 2014;103(1):35–41.
48. Hamada Y, et al. Histomorphometric analysis of diabetic osteopenia in streptozotocin-induced diabetic mice: a possible role of oxidative stress. Bone 2007;40(5):1408–14.
49. van der Kallen CJ, et al. Endoplasmic reticulum stress-induced apoptosis in the development of diabetes: is there a role for adipose tissue and liver? Apoptosis 2009;14(12):1424–34.
50. Hough FS, et al. Mechanisms in endocrinology: mechanisms and evaluation of bone fragility in type 1 diabetes mellitus. Eur J Endocrinol 2016;174(4):R127–38.
51. Baynes JW. Role of oxidative stress in development of complications in diabetes. Diabetes 1991;40(4):405–12.
52. Sroga GE, Wu PC, Vashishth D. Insulin-like growth factor 1, glycation and bone fragility: implications for fracture resistance of bone. PLoS One 2015;10(1):e0117046.
53. Hunt HB, et al. Altered tissue composition, microarchitecture, and mechanical performance in cancellous bone from men with type 2 diabetes mellitus. J Bone Miner Res 2019;34(7):1191–206.
54. Shah VN, et al. Bone mineral density at femoral neck and lumbar spine in adults with type 1 diabetes: a meta-analysis and review of the literature. Osteoporos Int 2017;28(9):2601–10.
55. Shanbhogue VV, et al. Bone geometry, volumetric density, microarchitecture, and estimated bone strength assessed by HR-pQCT in adult patients with type 1 diabetes mellitus. J Bone Miner Res 2015;30(12):2188–99.
56. Khan TS, Fraser LA. Type 1 diabetes and osteoporosis: from molecular pathways to bone phenotype. J Osteoporos 2015;2015:174186.
57. Zhukouskaya VV, et al. Bone health in type 1 diabetes: focus on evaluation and treatment in clinical practice. J Endocrinol Invest 2015;38(9):941–50.
58. Ivers RQ, et al. Diabetes and risk of fracture: The Blue Mountains Eye Study. Diabetes Care 2001;24(7):1198–203.
59. Kemink SA, et al. Osteopenia in insulin-dependent diabetes mellitus; prevalence and aspects of pathophysiology. J Endocrinol Invest 2000;23(5):295–303.
60. Gilmour J, et al. Type 1 diabetes and bone microarchitecture assessment with Trabecular Bone Score (TBS): a descriptive study. J Clin Densitom 2018;21(1):27.
61. Farlay D, et al. Nonenzymatic glycation and degree of mineralization are higher in bone from fractured patients with type 1 diabetes mellitus. J Bone Miner Res 2016;31(1):190–5.
62. Massé PG, et al. Bone metabolic abnormalities associated with well-controlled type 1 diabetes (IDDM) in young adult women: a disease complication often ignored or neglected. J Am Coll Nutr 2010;29(4):419–29.
63. McCabe LR. Understanding the pathology and mechanisms of type I diabetic bone loss. J Cell Biochem 2007;102(6):1343–57.
64. Kanazawa I, et al. Serum undercarboxylated osteocalcin was inversely associated with plasma glucose level and fat mass in type 2 diabetes mellitus. Osteoporos Int 2011;22(1):187–94.

65. Kanazawa I, et al. Serum osteocalcin level is associated with glucose metabolism and atherosclerosis parameters in type 2 diabetes mellitus. J Clin Endocrinol Metab 2009;94(1):45–9.

66. Neumann T, et al. Clinical and endocrine correlates of circulating sclerostin levels in patients with type 1 diabetes mellitus. Clin Endocrinol (Oxf) 2014;80(5):649–55.

67. van Bezooijen RL, et al. Wnt but not BMP signaling is involved in the inhibitory action of sclerostin on BMP-stimulated bone formation. J Bone Miner Res 2007; 22(1):19–28.

68. Hidayat K, et al. The use of metformin, insulin, sulphonylureas, and thiazolidine-diones and the risk of fracture: Systematic review and meta-analysis of observational studies. Obes Rev 2019;20(10):1494–503.

69. Jeyabalan J, et al. The anti-diabetic drug metformin does not affect bone mass in vivo or fracture healing. Osteoporos Int 2013;24(10):2659–70.

70. Vestergaard P, Rejnmark L, Mosekilde L. Relative fracture risk in patients with diabetes mellitus, and the impact of insulin and oral antidiabetic medication on relative fracture risk. Diabetologia 2005;48(7):1292–9.

71. Sofer E, Shargorodsky M. Effect of metformin treatment on circulating osteoprotegerin in patients with nonalcoholic fatty liver disease. Hepatol Int 2016;10(1): 169–74.

72. Lecka-Czernik B. Diabetes, bone and glucose-lowering agents: basic biology. Diabetologia 2017;60(7):1163–9.

73. Salari-Moghaddam A, et al. Metformin use and risk of fracture: a systematic review and meta-analysis of observational studies. Osteoporos Int 2019;30(6): 1167–73.

74. Kahn SE, et al. Rosiglitazone-associated fractures in type 2 diabetes: an Analysis from A Diabetes Outcome Progression Trial (ADOPT). Diabetes Care 2008;31(5): 845–51.

75. Oh TK, Song IA. Metformin therapy and hip fracture risk among patients with type II diabetes mellitus: a population-based cohort study. Bone 2020;135:115325.

76. Zhang Z, et al. Sulfonylurea and fracture risk in patients with type 2 diabetes mellitus: a meta-analysis. Diabetes Res Clin Pract 2020;159:107990.

77. Xie D, et al. Glucose-dependent insulinotropic peptide-overexpressing transgenic mice have increased bone mass. Bone 2007;40(5):1352–60.

78. Yamada C, et al. The murine glucagon-like peptide-1 receptor is essential for control of bone resorption. Endocrinology 2008;149(2):574–9.

79. Monami M, et al. Dipeptidyl peptidase-4 inhibitors and bone fractures: a meta-analysis of randomized clinical trials. Diabetes Care 2011;34(11):2474–6.

80. Cheng L, et al. Glucagon-like peptide-1 receptor agonists and risk of bone fracture in patients with type 2 diabetes: a meta-analysis of randomized controlled trials. Diabetes Metab Res Rev 2019;35(7):e3168.

81. Hidayat K, Du X, Shi BM. Risk of fracture with dipeptidyl peptidase-4 inhibitors, glucagon-like peptide-1 receptor agonists, or sodium-glucose cotransporter-2 inhibitors in real-world use: systematic review and meta-analysis of observational studies. Osteoporos Int 2019;30(10):1923–40.

82. Bilezikian JP, et al. Evaluation of bone mineral density and bone biomarkers in patients with type 2 diabetes treated with canagliflozin. J Clin Endocrinol Metab 2016;101(1):44–51.

83. Watts NB, et al. Effects of canagliflozin on fracture risk in patients with type 2 diabetes mellitus. J Clin Endocrinol Metab 2016;101(1):157–66.

84. Neal B, et al. Canagliflozin and cardiovascular and renal events in type 2 diabetes. N Engl J Med 2017;377(7):644–57.

85. Ruanpeng D, et al. Sodium-glucose cotransporter 2 (SGLT2) inhibitors and fracture risk in patients with type 2 diabetes mellitus: a meta-analysis. Diabetes Metab Res Rev 2017;33(6).
86. Azharuddin M, et al. Sodium-glucose cotransporter 2 inhibitors and fracture risk in patients with type 2 diabetes mellitus: a systematic literature review and Bayesian network meta-analysis of randomized controlled trials. Diabetes Res Clin Pract 2018;146:180–90.
87. Fralick M, et al. Fracture risk after initiation of use of canagliflozin: a cohort study. Ann Intern Med 2019;170(3):155–63.
88. Ueda P, et al. Sodium glucose cotransporter 2 inhibitors and risk of serious adverse events: nationwide register based cohort study. BMJ 2018;363:k4365.
89. Melton LJ 3rd, et al. Fracture risk in type 2 diabetes: update of a population-based study. J Bone Miner Res 2008;23(8):1334–42.
90. Thrailkill KM, et al. Is insulin an anabolic agent in bone? Dissecting the diabetic bone for clues. Am J Physiol Endocrinol Metab 2005;289(5):E735–45.
91. Pscherer S, et al. Fracture risk in patients with type 2 diabetes under different antidiabetic treatment regimens: a retrospective database analysis in primary care. Diabetes Metab Syndr Obes 2016;9:17–23.
92. Zhang Y, et al. Insulin use and fracture risk in patients with type 2 diabetes: a meta-analysis of 138,690 patients. Exp Ther Med 2019;17(5):3957–64.
93. Losada-Grande E, et al. Insulin use and excess fracture risk in patients with type 2 diabetes: a propensity-matched cohort analysis. Sci Rep 2017;7(1):3781.
94. Kennedy RL, et al. Accidents in patients with insulin-treated diabetes: increased risk of low-impact falls but not motor vehicle crashes–a prospective register-based study. J Trauma 2002;52(4):660–6.

Diabetes and Osteoporosis
Part II, Clinical Management

G. Isanne Schacter, MD, FRCPC[a], William D. Leslie, MD, FRCPC, MSc[b],*

KEYWORDS

- Diabetes • Bone • Osteoporosis • Fracture • Bone mineral density
- Dual-energy x-ray absorptiometry

KEY POINTS

- Risk assessment tools, including FRAX, are able to stratify fracture risk, but may underestimate the increased risk of fracture in diabetes mellitus without additional considerations.
- Bisphosphonates are the first line of treatment, although their efficacy in diabetes-induced osteoporosis is uncertain.
- The available data suggest that the presence of diabetes does not alter antiosteoporotic treatment response with regard to bone mineral density increase or fracture risk reduction.

BACKGROUND

Osteoporosis is a growing public health problem, with an impact on quality and quantity of life that crosses medical, social, and economic lines.[1] By the age of 50, the lifetime risk of hip fracture (HF) is approximately 17.5% for women and 6% for men in the United States.[2] The total number of HFs is projected to double by 2025 and double again by 2050.[3] As noted in part I of this review, both type 1 (T1D) and type 2 (T2D) diabetes mellitus are associated with an increased risk of osteoporotic fracture, especially HF, with much greater risk in the former.[4] There also appears to be a higher mortality after HF for individuals with diabetes.[5]

The 2020 American Association of Clinical Endocrinologists guidelines provide detailed recommendations on the evaluation and treatment of postmenopausal women with osteoporosis.[1] Individuals with diabetes are identified as a special population whereby these general recommendations may need to be adapted. Part II of this review examines considerations in the clinical management of individuals with diabetes-induced osteoporosis. A proposed approach to fracture risk evaluation

The authors have nothing to disclose.
[a] Department of Medicine, Rady Faculty of Health Sciences, University of Manitoba, GF-335, 820 Sherbrook Street, Winnipeg, Manitoba R3A 1R9, Canada; [b] Department of Medicine, Rady Faculty of Health Sciences, University of Manitoba, C5121, 409 Tache Avenue, Winnipeg, Manitoba R2H 2A6, Canada
* Corresponding author.
E-mail address: bleslie@sbgh.mb.ca

Endocrinol Metab Clin N Am 50 (2021) 287–297
https://doi.org/10.1016/j.ecl.2021.03.006
0889-8529/21/© 2021 Elsevier Inc. All rights reserved.

and treatment initiation in patients with diabetes from the International Osteoporosis Foundation is presented in **Fig. 1**[6] and incorporates diabetes-specific clinical risk and adjustments to fracture risk assessment.

FRACTURE RISK ASSESSMENT

Bone mineral density (BMD) is the most commonly reported measurement from dual-energy x-ray absorptiometry (DXA). However, other DXA-derived parameters for evaluating fracture risk are available and include skeletal geometry, trabecular bone score (TBS), vertebral fracture assessment (VFA), and body composition.

Bone Mineral Density

DXA measurement of BMD has traditionally been used to diagnose osteoporosis and assess risk of fracture. For each standard deviation (SD) decrease in BMD, fracture risk increases 1.4- to 2.6-fold.[7,8]

Patients with T1D have reduced BMD as compared with healthy controls.[4] A significant reduction in age-adjusted BMD (z score) is seen at both the hip (mean difference,

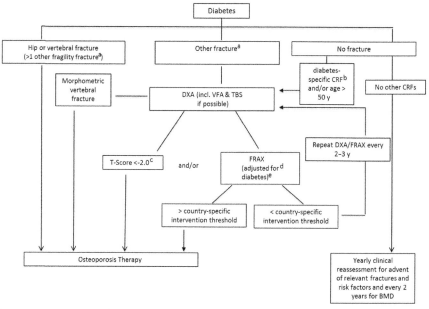

Fig. 1. Fracture risk evaluation in patients with diabetes (from the International Osteoporosis Foundation Bone and Diabetes Working Group). [a] In certain countries, humerus or pelvis fractures are also sufficient to initiate therapy; otherwise, more than nonvertebral nonhip fragility fracture could be required to initiate therapy. Alternatively, a nonvertebral nonhip fragility fracture should prompt further examinations to evaluate fracture risk. [b] Diabetes-specific clinical risk factors. [c] In diabetes, fracture risk at T score < −2 equivalent for nondiabetes at T score < −2.5. [d] Depending on country-specific guidelines for therapies. [e] For example, with TBS and/or "RA" = yes. CRF, clinical risk factor. (*From* Ferrari SL, Abrahamsen B, Napoli N, Akesson K, Chandran M, Eastell R, El-Hajj Fuleihan G, Josse R, Kendler DL, Kraenzlin M, Suzuki A, Pierroz DD, Schwartz AV, Leslie WD; Bone and Diabetes Working Group of IOF. Diagnosis and management of bone fragility in diabetes: an emerging challenge. Osteoporos Int. 2018;29(12):2585-2596; with permission.)

−0.37) and the lumbar spine (mean difference, −0.22). The reduction in BMD only partially explains the much higher HF risk when compared with individuals without diabetes.[4,9] There have not been adequately powered studies to examine the ability of BMD to predict fractures in T1D.

The effect of T2D on BMD has been inconsistent. Meta-analyses provide evidence for normal or paradoxically increased BMD at both the hip and the spine,[4] despite the increased fracture risk.[4,9] The observed increased risk for HF contrasts with an expected relative risk (RR) of 0.7 (ie, 30% lower risk) expected based on the degree of BMD elevation in T2D. Pooled results from 3 large prospective observational cohorts found that the fracture risk for any given femoral BMD T score and age was increased in patients with T2D as compared with normal controls.[10] Although age-adjusted hazard ratios (HRs) per SD decrease in BMD for HF and nonspine fracture were similar in patients with and without diabetes, at the same level of risk, mean femoral neck T score was approximately 0.59 (95% confidence interval [CI] 0.31–0.87) higher in women with T2D, and 0.38 (95% CI 0.09–0.66) higher in men with T2D.

In an observational registry-based study of 4218 subjects with 1 or more incident major osteoporotic fractures (MOF) (including 1108 with incident HFs), femoral neck BMD was significantly greater in those with diabetes ($P<.001$).[11] The adjusted HR per SD decrease in femoral neck T score was similar in those with and without diabetes (1.60, 95% CI: 1.44–1.79 vs 1.68; 95% CI: 1.61–1.75; P for interaction, .456). Each SD decrease in femoral neck T score strongly predicted HF in subjects with and without diabetes (HR, 2.15; 95% CI: 1.75–2.6 vs 2.17; 95% CI: 1.98–2.38; P for interaction, .956).

In summary, lower BMD is predictive of fractures in T2D, similar to the general population. However, the excess fracture risk in T2D is not captured by BMD, which is paradoxically higher. BMD can stratify fracture risk, but it does not account for differences between T2D and the general population.

Skeletal Geometry

Hip geometry measurements include hip structural analysis (HSA), hip axis length, and neck shaft angle.[12] Few studies have assessed geometric properties of bone strength in adults with T1D. Earlier age at onset of T1D has been found to be significantly associated with lower measures of bone strength in 1 study.[13] A second study did not demonstrate significantly different hip BMD or geometry from age-, weight-, and height-matched controls.[14] To date, there have been no studies of hip geometry in patients with T1D with fracture as the outcome. In a more recent study of 17 male T1D patients and 18 sex-matched health controls, Ishikawa and colleagues[15] found that the T1D patients had significantly lower cortical volumetric BMD (vBMD) in the femoral neck, and significantly lower total vBMD, cortical thickness, and cortical cross-sectional area (CSA) in the intertrochanter. Bone strength estimated by the buckling ratio (an index of cortical instability) of the intertrochanter was also significantly higher in the T1D patients.

Few studies have evaluated hip structure in T2D. Among 6000 postmenopausal women from the WHI-OS (Women's Health Initiative Observational Study), hip BMD and many HSA-derived measurements were higher in the 427 women with T2D, although differences disappeared after adjustment for other variables, including total lean body weight.[16] Hip CSA, section modulus, and BMD normalized to lean body mass were lower in women with T2D receiving insulin. A small cross-sectional study of 134 subjects with T2D not requiring insulin, lean mass (but not fat mass) was found to have a positive correlation with BMD and HSA-derived measurements (CSA, section modulus, and buckling ratio).[17] Another Canadian study of more than 3600 women (157 with T2D) used engineering beam theory and found that stresses were 4.5% higher in women with T2D as compared with controls (11.03 ± 0.18 megapascals (MPa) vs 10.56 ± 0.04 MPa; P = .0093), suggesting weaker geometry and an impaired skeletal load response in those with T2D.[18] SWAN (Study of Women's Health Across the Nation) enrolled more than 1800 women and found that even though women with T2D had a greater BMD at the femoral neck, they had lower composite indices for strength relative to load (−0.20 SD [95% CI: 0.38 to −0.03] for compression; −0.19 SD [95% CI: −0.38 to −0.003] for bending; and −0.19 SD [95% CI: −0.37 to −0.02] for impact).[19] An analysis of more than 1100 men (12.5% with T2D) found no association between T2D and HSA-based geometry measurements of strength.[20]

Trabecular Bone Score

TBS is a texture parameter derived from pixel-gray level variation in the spine DXA image, which predicts fracture risk independent of BMD.[21] This led to its implementation as an adjustment to the FRAX score[22] and subsequent validation in a multicohort meta-analysis.[23]

Sparse data exist on spine TBS in T1D. A cross-sectional study revealed a borderline reduction in mean TBS for T1D patients versus gender-, age- and body mass index (BMI)-matched controls (1.357 ± 0.129 vs 1.389 ± 0.085, respectively; P = .076).[24] T1D patients with prevalent fractures had significantly lower TBS as compared with T1D patients without fractures (1.309 ± 0.125 vs 1.370 ± 0.127; P = .04). TBS and hemoglobin A1c were independently associated with prevalent fractures. A TBS cutoff of less than 1.42 captured prevalent fractures with 91.7% sensitivity and 43.2% specificity. Only TBS and total hip BMD discriminated between patients with and without fractures (area under the curve [AUC] 0.63 [95% CI: 0.51–0.74; P = .48] and AUC 0.64 [95% CI: 0.51–0.78, P = .032], respectively). Lumbar spine TBS and total hip BMD in combination increased the AUC to 0.68 (95% CI: 0.55–0.81; P = .007).

A large clinical DXA registry analyzed results from almost 30,000 women (approximately 2300 with diabetes).[25] Diabetes was associated with higher BMD at all sites, whereas lumbar spine TBS was lower in both unadjusted and covariate-adjusted models (all P<.001). Lumbar spine TBS was an equally strong BMD-independent predictor of fracture in women with and without diabetes (adjusted HR, 1.27 [95% CI: 1.10–1.46] vs HR, 1.31 [95% CI: 1.24–1.38]). Lumbar spine TBS was found to partially explain the effect of diabetes on fracture risk in the prediction model. However, the opposite effect was seen when BMD measurements were added where the effect of diabetes was paradoxically increased. Ho-Pham and Nguyen[26] meta-analyzed 12 studies of 35,546 women and 4962 men aged 30 years or older. Patients with diabetes had significantly lower TBS than those without diabetes, with standardized mean difference being −0.31 (95% CI: −0.45 to −0.16), which was greater in women (−0.50; 95% CI: −0.69 to −0.32) than in men (−0.04; 95% CI: −0.17 to 0.10). In summary, TBS predicts fractures in postmenopausal women with and without diabetes. TBS scores in women with T2D are lower, and this partially accounts for the excess fracture risk in T2D.

Vertebral Fracture Assessment

VFA can be used to detect thoracic and lumbar spine vertebral fractures,[27] which in turn increase the risk of both vertebral and nonvertebral fractures independent of age, BMD, and baseline fracture probability from FRAX.[28,29] There is limited evidence for the use of VFA for fracture risk prediction in T1D. One small cross-sectional study demonstrated a higher prevalence of vertebral fractures when compared with controls (24.4 vs 6.1%; P = .002).[30] There are no published studies assessing VFA in T2D. VFA image quality is degraded in obese patients, which may affect test performance in patients with T2D.

Body Composition

Sarcopenia (reduced appendicular muscle mass and function) commonly occurs later in life and is a potential risk factor for fracture.[31] DXA is a well-validated technique for analyzing body composition, muscle, and fat mass[32] and can also be used to estimate visceral adipose tissue (VAT). VAT is a metabolically active pathogenic fat depot that has been implicated in insulin resistance and T2D and has also been shown to be a risk factor for fracture.[33,34]

There are no adult studies examining the role of body composition on fracture risk in T1D. Studies in children with T1D have demonstrated lower lean body mass but greater total fat mass, abdominal fat percentage, soft tissue fat mass percentage, and fat/lean ratio.[35]

Body composition, and more specifically abdominal adiposity, is strongly associated with metabolic disorders, including T2D, and may have a causal role in their development.[35] Intraabdominal fat is closely linked to the metabolic syndrome and T2D.[36,37] There was a strong positive association demonstrated between VAT and T2D in a cross-sectional analysis of more than 900 subjects.[38] Multivariable regression analysis revealed that DXA VAT was significantly associated with increased odds of cardiometabolic indicators, including impaired fasting glucose and T2D. After adjustment for BMI and waist circumference, the odds ratio per SD increase in VAT for T2D was 2.97 (95% CI: 0.73–5.87) in women and 2.25 (95% CI: 1.21–4.19) in men. A longitudinal cohort study in 30,252 women found that abdominal fat from spine DXA (but not hip fat) was strongly associated with newly diagnosed diabetes in those without diabetes at baseline, and this risk was independent of age, BMI, and comorbidities (adjusted HR, 3.56; 95% CI: 2.67–4.75 highest vs lowest quintile).[39] Another study demonstrated that men with T2D have lower muscle mass and strength than nondiabetic controls.[20] These differences in nonskeletal factors were thought to at least partially explain the greater incidence in falls and fractures in patients with T2D. There are currently no studies examining whether either body composition, VAT, or sarcopenia is a predictor of fracture in T2D.

Fracture Prediction Tools

Several validated fracture prediction tools can assess fracture risk in the general population: the fracture risk assessment tool (FRAX; available: www.shef.ac.uk/FRAX/index.aspx), the Garvan fracture risk calculator (available: www.garvan.org.au/bone-fracture-risk), and the QFracture score (available: www.qfracture.org/). Only the QFracture score has specific inputs for T1D and T2D.[40] No studies have evaluated the Garvan calculator in subjects with either T1D or T2D, but because the calculator includes falls, it may capture some of the diabetes-associated risk.

The FRAX tool is based on easily assessed risk factors identified in meta-analyses of population-based prospective cohorts.[41] T1D is not presented as a primary entry variable in the FRAX algorithm but is considered under secondary osteoporosis. As such, it is given the same weight as rheumatoid arthritis (RA; the prototype for all causes of secondary osteoporosis). Coding secondary osteoporosis only increases fracture probability when BMD is not included in the FRAX calculation.[42] Including secondary osteoporosis or BMD in the FRAX calculation may partially account for the excess risk for MOFs in T1D but would not account for the very high risk for HFs. There are no studies directly assessing the performance of FRAX (with or without BMD) for predicting fracture risk in T1D.

Studies have shown that FRAX underestimates the actual observed risk of fracture in T2D.[10,43] In 3 combined prospective observational cohorts comprising greater than 9500 women and 7400 men, for a given FRAX probability, both women and men with T2D had a higher observed fracture risk.[10] FRAX was found to stratify hip and non-spine fracture risk equally well in those with and without diabetes (all P for interaction, >.10), despite the higher fracture risk attributable to T2D. In a study of more than 3500 older patients with predominantly T2D from a large clinical registry, diabetes was found to be a risk factor for subsequent MOF (adjusted HR, 1.61; 95% CI: 1.42–1.83) and HF (adjusted HR, 6.27; 95% CI: 3.62–10.87 aged <65 years; 95% CI: 1.71–2.90 aged ≥65 years).[43] FRAX was able to stratify fracture risk in those with diabetes (AUC for MOF 0.67; 95% CI: 0.63–0.70; AUC for HF 0.77; 95% CI: 0.72–081) only slightly less well than in those without diabetes. However, FRAX again underestimated cumulative observed MOF and HF risk in subjects with diabetes, even after accounting for mortality differences.

A subsequent analysis from the same database of 62,000 individuals aged 40 years and older (10% with diabetes) showed that diabetes and the FRAX risk factors were independently associated with MOFs and HFs.[11] Importantly, diabetes did not modify the effect of individual risk factors on subsequent MOF: 10-year increase in age in those without and with diabetes (HR, 1.43 vs HR, 1.39; P for interaction, .781), RA (1.43 vs 1.74; P for interaction, .325), and prior fracture (1.62 vs 1.72; P for interaction, .588) when adjusted for BMD. After excluding BMD, an increase in BMI of 5 kg/m^2 was similarly protective against MOF in those without and with diabetes (HR, 0.83 vs 0.79; P for interaction, .276). For HF, age had a weaker effect in those with versus those without diabetes (P for interaction, <.001).

In summary, FRAX provides similar fracture discrimination in the diabetes and general populations; however, absolute fracture risk is underestimated. The lack of significant interactions between diabetes and FRAX risk factors or FRAX scores for predicting MOF implies the potential for modifying the existing FRAX tool to accommodate the unmeasured effect of T2D. Several methods have been proposed to act as proxy for T2D given its absence as an input variable in FRAX. Leslie and colleagues[44] directly compared 4 proposed methods to improve the performance of FRAX for T2D by (1) including the RA input to FRAX; (2) making a TBS adjustment to FRAX; (3) reducing the femoral neck T-score input to FRAX by 0.5 SD; and (4) increasing the age input to FRAX by 10 years. Incident MOFs and HFs were ascertained over a mean of 8.3 years among 44,543 women and men 40 years of age or older (4136 with diabetes). All 4 FRAX adjustments attenuated the effect of diabetes, but a residual effect of diabetes was seen on MOF risk after TBS adjustment, and on HF risk after the RA and TBS adjustments. For those with diabetes, the unadjusted FRAX risk underestimated MOF (observed/predicted ratio, 1.15; 95% CI: 1.03–1.28), but this was no longer significant after applying any of the diabetes adjustments. HF risk was more severely underestimated (observed/predicted ratio 1.85; 95% CI: 1.51–2.20) and was only partially corrected with the diabetes adjustments (still significant for the RA and TBS adjustments). Among those with diabetes, there was moderate reclassification based on a fixed MOF cutoff of 20% (4.1% to 7.1%) or fixed HF cutoff of 3% (5.7% to 16.5%). Net reclassification improvement increased for MOF with each of the diabetes adjustments (range, 3.9% to 5.6% in the diabetes subgroup). Ultimately, each of the proposed methods for addressing limitations in the ability of FRAX to assess fracture risk in individuals with diabetes was found to improve performance, although no single method was optimal in all settings.

MANAGEMENT

Antiresorptive agents are currently the first-line therapy for antiosteoporosis treatment.[1,45] Selecting an agent with demonstrated efficacy for HF prevention is important given the particularly high risk for HFs in T1D and T2D. Antiresorptive agents decrease osteoclast activity and slow bone turnover, allowing for a modest gain in BMD with stabilization in skeletal microstructure, which in turn leads to a reduced fracture risk.[46] However, if bone is already deficient in osteoblast function, then antiresorptive agents may be less effective. Evidence exists that high bone turnover in comparison with low bone turnover at baseline significantly predicts greater response to bisphosphonate treatment.[47] Anabolic agents have been increasingly used in treatment of those at very high fracture risk. Animal trials demonstrated that use of intermittent parenteral parathyroid hormone analogue (teriparatide) increased osteoblast survival with a decrease in diabetes-associated bone loss.[48] However, there has also been a demonstrated significant increase in cortical porosity seen with teriparatide monotherapy that has not been noted with denosumab, either alone or in combination with teriparitide.[49] Romosozumab, a new monoclonal antibody that binds sclerostin, increases bone formation and decreases bone resorption.

A network meta-analysis by Barrionuevo and colleagues[45] provides comparative effective estimates for the various available treatments to reduce the risk of fragility fractures in postmenopausal women. Very little information is available from comparative studies on the effectiveness of osteoporosis treatment in diabetes in general, and particularly in T1D. This has been compounded by the fact that diabetes is often an exclusion criterion for enrollment in clinical trials.

The FIT (Fracture Intervention Trial) involving 6450 women aged 54 to 81 years with low femoral neck BMD demonstrated an increase in BMD at all sites (6.6% at the lumbar spine and 2.4% at the hip) in diabetes patients treated with alendronate for 3 years.[50] Similar results were found in subjects without diabetes and contrasted with subjects with diabetes in the placebo group, who lost more BMD at the total hip as compared with subjects without diabetes. Women with and without diabetes also experienced similar decreases in markers of bone turnover. Although the investigators concluded that antiresorptive therapy was as effective in T2D as in those without diabetes, the study was underpowered to compare fracture outcomes. There currently are no studies analyzing the response to romosozumab in patients with diabetes.

A recent systematic review by Anagnostis and colleagues[51] analyzed 5 studies comprising 9 subjects, primarily with T2D. Alendronate demonstrated comparable vertebral antifracture efficacy in patients with and without diabetes (n = 2), whereas nonvertebral fracture risk was either the same (n = 1) or higher in diabetic patients (n = 1). Teriparatide (n = 1) demonstrated the same nonvertebral fracture rates in both patients with and without T2D. Regarding BMD, equal increases in spine BMD were observed with alendronate (n = 4), risedronate (n = 1), and teriparatide (n = 1). With respect to hip BMD, similar increases were observed with teriparatide (n = 1), whereas data regarding alendronate were controversial (n = 3). The investigators concluded that the presence of diabetes does not alter antiosteoporotic treatment response, regarding BMD increase or vertebral fracture risk reduction.

Ferrari and colleagues[52] performed a post hoc analysis of the 3-year, placebo-controlled FREEDOM study and 7-year extension. Of 7808 postmenopausal women in FREEDOM, 508 with diabetes received denosumab (n = 266) or placebo (n = 242). BMD increased significantly in subjects with T2D with denosumab versus placebo in FREEDOM and continued to increase during the extension in long-term (continuing denosumab) and crossover (placebo to denosumab) subjects. Denosumab-treated subjects with diabetes had significantly lower new vertebral fracture rates (1.6%) versus placebo (8.0%) (RR 0.20; 95% CI: 0.07–0.61; P = .001). Nonvertebral fracture incidence was higher with denosumab (11.7%) versus placebo (5.9%) (HR, 1.94; 95% CI: 1.00–3.77; P = .046), although there were slightly fewer HFs with denosumab (1 vs 4; nonsignificant). Overall, denosumab significantly increased BMD and decreased vertebral fracture risk in subjects with osteoporosis and diabetes. No reduction in nonvertebral fractures was observed.

Dhaliwal and colleagues[53] analyzed patients with T2D from ACTIVE (Abaloparatide Comparator Trial In Vertebral Endpoints), a phase 3, double-blind, randomized, placebo- and active-controlled trial of a total of 198 women with postmenopausal osteoporosis and T2D from 21 centers in 10 countries. Participants were randomized 1:1:1 to daily subcutaneous injections of placebo, abaloparatide (80 µg), or open-label teriparatide (20 µg) for 18 months. Significant (P<.001) improvements in BMD at the total hip (mean change, 3.0% vs −0.4%), femoral neck (2.6% vs −0.2%), lumbar spine (8.9% vs 1.3%), and TBS at lumbar spine (3.72% vs −0.56%) were observed with abaloparatide versus placebo at 18 months. Despite the small number of subjects and fracture events, significantly fewer nonvertebral fractures were seen in patients with T2D treated with abaloparatide versus placebo (P = .04).

SUMMARY

Diabetes-induced osteoporosis in both T1D and T2D is characterized by an increase in fracture risk. Several fracture risk assessment tools are available to help stratify fracture risk. FRAX, the most widely used tool, only partially captures the excess risk in T1D and also underestimates the risk in T2D. Although BMD from DXA and FRAX is still useful clinically and stratifies fracture risk in those with diabetes, recent enhancements can help to better identify those at increased risk of fracture. Incorporating this additional information into risk prediction may help to identify subjects with diabetes who are at high risk for fracture and in whom treatment is most likely to be beneficial. The available data suggest that the presence of diabetes does not alter antiosteoporotic treatment response.

CLINICS CARE POINTS

- There are no studies directly assessing the performance of FRAX (with or without BMD) for predicting fracture risk in T1D.
- Individual FRAX risk factors (including BMD) remain important in patients with T2D. FRAX provides similar fracture discrimination in the diabetes and general populations; however, absolute fracture risk is underestimated. Several methods have been developed to capture the risk associated with T2D given its absence as an input variable in FRAX.
- Antiresorptive agents are currently the first-line therapy for antiosteoporosis treatment, although anabolic agents may be preferred in those at very high fracture risk. Selecting an agent with demonstrated efficacy for hip fracture prevention is important given the particularly high risk for hip fractures in T1D and T2D.

REFERENCES

1. Camacho PM, et al. American Association of Clinical Endocrinologists/American College of Endocrinology clinical practice guidelines for the diagnosis and

treatment of postmenopausal osteoporosis-2020 update. Endocr Pract 2020; 26(Suppl 1):1–46.

2. Melton LJ 3rd, et al. How many women have osteoporosis? JBMR Anniversary Classic. JBMR, Volume 7, Number 9, 1992. J Bone Miner Res 2005;20(5):886–92.

3. Gullberg B, Johnell O, Kanis JA. World-wide projections for hip fracture. Osteoporos Int 1997;7(5):407–13.

4. Vestergaard P. Discrepancies in bone mineral density and fracture risk in patients with type 1 and type 2 diabetes–a meta-analysis. Osteoporos Int 2007;18(4): 427–44.

5. Tebe C, et al. The association between type 2 diabetes mellitus, hip fracture, and post-hip fracture mortality: a multi-state cohort analysis. Osteoporos Int 2019; 30(12):2407–15.

6. Ferrari SL, et al. Diagnosis and management of bone fragility in diabetes: an emerging challenge. Osteoporos Int 2018;29(12):2585–96.

7. Johnell O, et al. Predictive value of BMD for hip and other fractures. J Bone Miner Res 2005;20(7):1185–94.

8. Marshall D, Johnell O, Wedel H. Meta-analysis of how well measures of bone mineral density predict occurrence of osteoporotic fractures. BMJ 1996;312(7041): 1254–9.

9. Janghorbani M, et al. Systematic review of type 1 and type 2 diabetes mellitus and risk of fracture. Am J Epidemiol 2007;166(5):495–505.

10. Schwartz AV, et al. Association of BMD and FRAX score with risk of fracture in older adults with type 2 diabetes. JAMA 2011;305(21):2184–92.

11. Leslie WD, et al. Does diabetes modify the effect of FRAX risk factors for predicting major osteoporotic and hip fracture? Osteoporos Int 2014;25(12):2817–24.

12. Broy SB, et al. Fracture risk prediction by non-BMD DXA measures: the 2015 ISCD Official Positions Part 1: hip geometry. J Clin Densitom 2015;18(3):287–308.

13. Maser RE, et al. Hip strength in adults with type 1 diabetes is associated with age at onset of diabetes. J Clin Densitom 2012;15(1):78–85.

14. Miazgowski T, et al. Bone mineral density and hip structural analysis in type 1 diabetic men. Eur J Endocrinol 2007;156(1):123–7.

15. Ishikawa K, et al. Type 1 diabetes patients have lower strength in femoral bone determined by quantitative computed tomography: a cross-sectional study. J Diabetes Investig 2015;6(6):726–33.

16. Garg R, et al. Hip geometry in diabetic women: implications for fracture risk. Metabolism 2012;61(12):1756–62.

17. Moseley KF, et al. Lean mass predicts hip geometry in men and women with non-insulin-requiring type 2 diabetes mellitus. J Clin Densitom 2011;14(3):332–9.

18. Hamilton CJ, et al. Evidence for impaired skeletal load adaptation among Canadian women with type 2 diabetes mellitus: insight into the BMD and bone fragility paradox. Metabolism 2013;62(10):1401–5.

19. Ishii S, et al. Diabetes and femoral neck strength: findings from the hip strength across the menopausal transition study. J Clin Endocrinol Metab 2012;97(1): 190–7.

20. Akeroyd JM, et al. Differences in skeletal and non-skeletal factors in a diverse sample of men with and without type 2 diabetes mellitus. J Diabet Complications 2014;28(5):679–83.

21. Martineau P, Leslie WD. The utility and limitations of using trabecular bone score with FRAX. Curr Opin Rheumatol 2018;30(4):412–9.

22. McCloskey EV, et al. Adjusting fracture probability by trabecular bone score. Calcif Tissue Int 2015;96(6):500–9.

23. McCloskey EV, et al. A meta-analysis of trabecular bone score in fracture risk prediction and its relationship to FRAX. J Bone Miner Res 2016;31(5):940–8.

24. Neumann T, et al. Trabecular bone score in type 1 diabetes–a cross-sectional study. Osteoporos Int 2016;27(1):127–33.

25. Leslie WD, et al. TBS (trabecular bone score) and diabetes-related fracture risk. J Clin Endocrinol Metab 2013;98(2):602–9.

26. Ho-Pham LT, Nguyen TV. Association between trabecular bone score and type 2 diabetes: a quantitative update of evidence. Osteoporos Int 2019;30(10): 2079–85.

27. Rosen HN, et al. The Official Positions of the International Society for Clinical Densitometry: vertebral fracture assessment. J Clin Densitom 2013;16(4):482–8.

28. Crans GG, Genant HK, Krege JH. Prognostic utility of a semiquantitative spinal deformity index. Bone 2005;37(2):175–9.

29. Schousboe JT, et al. Prevalent vertebral fracture on bone density lateral spine (VFA) images in routine clinical practice predict incident fractures. Bone 2019; 121:72–9.

30. Zhukouskaya VV, et al. Prevalence of morphometric vertebral fractures in patients with type 1 diabetes. Diabetes Care 2013;36(6):1635–40.

31. Binkley N, Cooper C. Sarcopenia, the next frontier in fracture prevention: introduction from the guest editors. J Clin Densitom 2015;18(4):459–60.

32. Albanese CV, Diessel E, Genant HK. Clinical applications of body composition measurements using DXA. J Clin Densitom 2003;6(2):75–85.

33. Meyer HE, et al. Abdominal obesity and hip fracture: results from the Nurses' Health Study and the Health Professionals Follow-Up Study. Osteoporos Int 2016;27(6):2127–36.

34. Yang S, et al. Association between abdominal obesity and fracture risk: a prospective study. J Clin Endocrinol Metab 2013;98(6):2478–83.

35. Abd El Dayem SM, et al. Bone density, body composition, and markers of bone remodeling in type 1 diabetic patients. Scand J Clin Lab Invest 2011;71(5): 387–93.

36. von Eyben FE, et al. Intra-abdominal obesity and metabolic risk factors: a study of young adults. Int J Obes Relat Metab Disord 2003;27(8):941–9.

37. Jensen MD. Role of body fat distribution and the metabolic complications of obesity. J Clin Endocrinol Metab 2008;93(11 Suppl 1):S57–63.

38. Rothney MP, et al. Abdominal visceral fat measurement using dual-energy X-ray: association with cardiometabolic risk factors. Obesity (Silver Spring) 2013;21(9): 1798–802.

39. Leslie WD, Ludwig SM, Morin S. Abdominal fat from spine dual-energy x-ray absorptiometry and risk for subsequent diabetes. J Clin Endocrinol Metab 2010; 95(7):3272–6.

40. Leslie WD. Fracture risk assessment in diabetes. In: Lecka-Czernik B, Fowlkes JL, editors. Diabetic bone disease. Switzerland: Springer International; 2016. p. 45–69.

41. Kanis JA, on behalf of the World Health Organization Scientific Group. Assessment of osteoporosis at the primary health-care level. Technical Report. United Kingdom: WHO Collaborating Centre, Univeristy of Sheffield; 2008.

42. Hough FS, et al. Mechanisms in endocrinology: mechanisms and evaluation of bone fragility in type 1 diabetes mellitus. Eur J Endocrinol 2016;174(4):R127–38.

43. Giangregorio LM, et al. FRAX underestimates fracture risk in patients with diabetes. J Bone Miner Res 2012;27(2):301–8.

44. Leslie WD, et al. Comparison of methods for improving fracture risk assessment in diabetes: the Manitoba BMD registry. J Bone Miner Res 2018;33(11):1923–30.
45. Barrionuevo P, et al. Efficacy of pharmacological therapies for the prevention of fractures in postmenopausal women: a network meta-analysis. J Clin Endocrinol Metab 2019;104(5):1623–30.
46. Black DM, Rosen CJ. Postmenopausal osteoporosis. N Engl J Med 2016;374(21): 2096–7.
47. Gonnelli S, et al. Bone turnover and the response to alendronate treatment in postmenopausal osteoporosis. Calcif Tissue Int 1999;65(5):359–64.
48. Motyl KJ, McCauley LK, McCabe LR. Amelioration of type I diabetes-induced osteoporosis by parathyroid hormone is associated with improved osteoblast survival. J Cell Physiol 2012;227(4):1326–34.
49. Tsai JN, et al. Effects of two years of teriparatide, denosumab, or both on bone microarchitecture and strength (DATA-HRpQCT study). J Clin Endocrinol Metab 2016;101(5):2023–30.
50. Keegan TH, et al. Effect of alendronate on bone mineral density and biochemical markers of bone turnover in type 2 diabetic women: the Fracture Intervention Trial. Diabetes Care 2004;27(7):1547–53.
51. Anagnostis P, et al. Efficacy of anti-osteoporotic medications in patients with type 1 and 2 diabetes mellitus: a systematic review. Endocrine 2018;60(3):373–83.
52. Ferrari S, et al. Denosumab in postmenopausal women with osteoporosis and diabetes: subgroup analysis of FREEDOM and FREEDOM extension. Bone 2020;134:115268.
53. Dhaliwal R, et al. Abaloparatide in postmenopausal women with osteoporosis and type 2 diabetes: a post hoc analysis of the ACTIVE study. JBMR Plus 2020;4(4): e10346.

Assessment of Skeletal Strength

Bone Density Testing and Beyond

E. Michael Lewiecki, MD

KEYWORDS

- Osteoporosis • DXA • FRAX • TBS • HR-pQCT • FEA • PEUS • BCT

KEY POINTS

- Bone strength is determined by properties that include bone mineral density (BMD), architecture, and material properties.
- Dual-energy X-ray absorptiometry (DXA) is a commonly used technology to measure areal BMD and bone geometry, assess fracture risk, and monitor longitudinal changes in BMD.
- Fracture risk algorithms that include clinical risk factors for fracture predict fracture risk better than DXA or clinical risk factors alone.
- Advanced imaging technologies can measure volumetric BMD, assess bone microarchitecture, and provide input for mathematical models to predict the force required for a fracture.
- Minimally invasive procedures have been developed to provide in vivo assessment of bone material properties.

Measure what is measurable, and make measurable what is not so.
—Antoine-Augustin Cournot and Thomas-Henri Martin; often misattributed to
Galileo Galilei[1]

INTRODUCTION

Osteoporosis is defined as a skeletal disorder characterized by compromised bone strength predisposing a person to an increased risk of fracture.[2] Bone strength is determined by bone mineral density (BMD) and non-BMD skeletal properties that include geometry (eg, size and shape), microarchitecture (eg, internal structure of trabecular and cortical bone compartments), turnover (eg, magnitude and balance

Ethical Statement: The author is accountable for all aspects of the work in ensuring that questions related to accuracy or integrity of any part of the work are appropriately investigated and resolved.

New Mexico Clinical Research & Osteoporosis Center, 300 Oak Street Northeast, Albuquerque, NM 87106, USA

E-mail address: mlewiecki@gmail.com

Endocrinol Metab Clin N Am 50 (2021) 299–317
https://doi.org/10.1016/j.ecl.2021.03.008
0889-8529/21/© 2021 Elsevier Inc. All rights reserved.

endo.theclinics.com

of bone resorption and formation), damage accumulation (eg, microfractures), and tissue material properties. A bone fracture occurs when the load applied to a bone exceeds its strength, as when a sideways fall results in a hip fracture.

This review focuses on the clinical applications of commonly available technologies to assess skeletal strength and offers a glimpse at some technologies used in the research setting that have the potential for clinical use in the future. Appropriate use of these technologies may contribute to a reduction in the global burden of osteoporotic fractures and mitigate the serious personal consequences and high societal costs of fractures.[3]

BONE DENSITY TESTING
Dual-Energy X-ray Absorptiometry

Dual-energy X-ray absorptiometry (DXA) is the primary clinical tool for diagnosing osteoporosis, assessing fracture risk, and monitoring longitudinal changes in BMD.[4] Non-BMD skeletal applications of DXA include vertebral fracture assessment (VFA),[5] trabecular bone score (TBS),[6] and hip geometry.[7] DXA also can be used for non-BMD nonskeletal measurements such as abdominal aortic calcification[8] and analysis of body composition.[9] There is a correlation between BMD measured by DXA and bone strength in biomechanical studies of failure load in cadavers.[10] Lower BMD is associated with greater risk of fractures, with an approximate doubling in the relative risk of fracture for every 1 standard deviation decrease in BMD; this is similar or better than the predictive ability of blood pressure for stroke and better than serum cholesterol concentration for predicting cardiovascular disease.[11] Low BMD is typically one of the criteria for selecting patients for clinical trials of medications to reduce fracture risk.[12] The magnitude of BMD increase with osteoporosis treatment is highly correlated with reduction of fracture risk.[13] The accuracy and precision of DXA are excellent[14] and radiation exposure is low.[15]

A central DXA system is one that is capable of measuring BMD at the lumbar spine and hip ("central" skeletal sites) and sometimes the forearm, distal femur, and proximal tibia ("peripheral" skeletal sites). The test is performed with the patient supported by a table with an X-ray tube below and a photon detector above. The photon flux emitted by the X-ray tube is modified or filtered to produce 2 distinct photoelectric peaks that are attenuated differently when passing through the patient's bone and soft tissue. The intensities of the photon beams are recognized by a detector located on a movable arm above the table and analyzed by a computer that provides a quantitative measurement of BMD.[16] DXA measures bone mineral content in grams (g) and bone area in square centimeters (cm^2) to calculate areal BMD in g/cm^2. This is a 2-dimensional (2-D) projection of a three-dimensional (3-D) structure. A peripheral DXA (pDXA) device uses the same technology in a smaller more portable instrument that is dedicated to measuring BMD at peripheral skeletal sites, such as the forearm or calcaneus.[17]

BMD is used for quantitative comparison of serial measurements according to standards established by the International Society for Clinical Densitometry (ISCD).[18,19] To distinguish between a BMD change that is within the range of error and a statistically significant change, the reproducibility of the measurements must be assessed with in vivo precision assessment. This allows calculation of the least significant change, the smallest change in BMD that is statistically significant with a 95% level of confidence.

T-score is an expression of BMD that is used for diagnostic classification according to criteria established by the World Health Organization.[20] A T-score of −2.5 or below at the lumbar spine, femoral neck, total proximal femur, or 33% (one-third) radius in a postmenopausal woman or man age 50 years or older is consistent with a diagnosis of osteoporosis. However, it is important to recognize that a patient may have a T-score in this range and not have osteoporosis, such as when there is osteomalacia, and a patient may have a T-score better than −2.5 and have osteoporosis, such as when a fragility fracture has occurred.

Despite the many benefits of DXA in the evaluation of patients with skeletal disorders, there are concerns regarding the quality of the test at some facilities[21] and its underutilization,[22] which may be contributing to the global osteoporosis treatment gap[23] and an increase in fracture rates that has been observed in the United States.[24] Unmet needs in the care of patients with osteoporosis have led to consideration of other technologies to assess bone strength and fracture risk.

Quantitative Computed Tomography

Conventional computed tomography (CT) scanners with appropriate software can be used to measure volumetric BMD (vBMD) in milligrams per cubic centimeter (mg/cm³), with the capability of generating separate measurements of the trabecular and cortical bone compartments. This provides information not available with DXA and can exclude confounding effects of degenerative disease in the posterior elements of the spine that are common in older patients. CT scans done for any reason also provide an opportunity to identify previously unrecognized vertebral fractures.[25] Quantitative CT (QCT) skeletal measurements can be obtained intentionally or incidentally ("opportunistically") when a CT scan is obtained for diagnostic evaluation of a nonskeletal disorder.[26] Because more than 10% of the Medicare population in the United States has a CT scan of the pelvis or abdomen each year,[27] which is almost twice as many as are being screened for osteoporosis by DXA,[28] there are occasions for opportunistic QCT measurements that might identify patients at risk for fracture who are not otherwise recognized. Peripheral QCT (pQCT) devices use the same technology as QCT to measure vBMD at appendicular skeletal sites, such as the distal forearm or distal. Although the radiation exposure is lower than QCT and the cost is less, the relevance of pQCT in clinical practice is not well established. QCT has been helpful in the research setting to provide a better understanding of the structural changes occurring with skeletal diseases and the effects of pharmacologic agents intended to improve bone strength and reduce fracture risk.

vBMD measurements by QCT can be made with or without the use of a calibration phantom. A calibration phantom, typically containing a known density equivalent of potassium phosphate or hydroxyapatite, can be placed under the patient during the scan. The correlation between the attenuation of X-rays passing through bone and the known density of the phantom can then be established. Attenuation is usually expressed as Hounsfield Units (HU), which are normalized such that −1000 corresponds to air, 0 corresponds to water at standard temperature and pressure, and values >0 correspond to body tissue such as muscle and bone.[29] Practice parameters established by the American College of Radiology (ACR) state that phantom-based QCT acquisition can be done by simultaneous or asynchronous (ie, at different times) scanning of the phantom using manufacturer-specific techniques.[30] Asynchronous calibration assumes that the scanner provides stable results over time and good correlation with synchronous calibration. Phantomless calibration can be "tissue-based," whereby air, fat, muscle, and very dense cortical bone are assumed to have known density and linear attenuation values; or "blind" using previously defined HU/density relationships.[29] Asynchronous and phantomless techniques have been reported to have greater error than synchronous calibration,[29] but still are suitable for clinical applications, allowing for the development of opportunistic BMD testing when the CT scan was originally obtained for other reasons without inclusion of a phantom.

Two-dimensional areal BMD values and T-scores can be derived from 3-D QCT. QCT-derived T-scores at the femoral neck and total proximal femur are equivalent to DXA T-scores and can be used with the World Health Organization (WHO) diagnostic criteria.[19] QCT-derived femoral neck BMD with the Mindways QCT system (Mindways Software, Austin, TX) is an approved input for the FRAX fracture risk algorithm.[31] Total femur trabecular BMD by QCT predicts hip fracture risk as well as hip BMD measured by DXA. There are no consensus standards for diagnostic classification with spine QCT measurements, although the ACR suggests that trabecular spine vBMD values approximate the WHO diagnostic categories, as follows: osteoporosis for vBMD less than 80 mg/cm^3, osteopenia for vBMD 80 to 120 mg/cm^3, and normal for vBMD greater than 120 mg/cm^3.[30] Because QCT involves a higher dose of radiation and greater cost than DXA, the ISCD recommends using DXA rather than QCT when it is available and comparable information can be obtained. DXA-derived 3-D analysis of cortical and trabecular bone compartments has been studied with 3D-SHAPER software (Galgo Medical, Barcelona, Spain),[32] which has the potential of providing additional information on bone strength and fracture risk with low radiation exposure. When DXA cannot be done, treatment decisions may be made according to QCT measurements.

ULTRASOUND MEASUREMENTS
Quantitative Ultrasound

Quantitative ultrasound (QUS) is a technique for assessing bone strength at peripheral skeletal sites such as the calcaneus and forearm. It is inexpensive, portable, and does not involve ionizing radiation. Although QUS does not measure BMD, measurements at the calcaneus with validated devices can predict fracture risk in postmenopausal women and elderly men.[33,34] QUS T-scores may be reported, but these are not the same as DXA T-scores and cannot be used to diagnose osteoporosis according to the WHO criteria. The correlation between QUS T-scores and DXA T-scores is poor because of differences in skeletal sites and regions of interest, differences in technology, and the use of different reference databases.[24,25] QUS is not clinically useful for monitoring the skeletal effect of treatment because measured changes are too small and too slow to be helpful in making treatment decisions.

QUS devices produce inaudible high-frequency sound waves in the ultrasonic range, typically between 0.1 and 1.0 MHz. These are produced and detected by means of high-efficiency piezoelectric transducers. Acoustical contact with the skin can be achieved with a water bath, or by means of silicone pads or ultrasound gel, or a combination of these methods. There are substantial technical differences among QUS devices, which use variable frequencies, different transducer sizes, and sometimes measure different regions of interest, even at the same skeletal site. The calcaneus is the skeletal site most often tested, although other bones, including the radius, tibia, and finger phalanges, can be used. Two measurements are typically made: speed of sound (SOS) and broadband ultrasound attenuation (BUA). Proprietary device-specific values such "quantitative ultrasound index" and "stiffness index" may be derived from a combination of these measurements. SOS varies according to the type of bone, with a typical range of 3000 to 3600 m/s with cortical bone and 1650 to 2300 m/s for trabecular bone.[22] A higher SOS is associated with higher bone density. BUA, reported as decibels per megahertz (dB/MHz), is a measurement of the loss of energy (attenuation) of the sound wave as it passes through bone. As with SOS, a higher BUA is associated with higher bone density.

Pulse-Echo Ultrasound

Pulse-echo ultrasonography (PEUS) with the Bindex device (Bone Index Finland, Ltd, Kuopio, Finland) uses ultrasound to estimate the thickness of cortical bone at peripheral skeletal sites with a handheld device connected to a personal computer.[35] Ultrasonic waves with a frequency of 3.0 MHz are generated by a transducer that is placed on the skin overlying a peripheral skeletal site, such as the proximal tibia (**Fig. 1**). The lag time of pulsed waves reflected from the periosteal and endosteal surfaces is measured, with a longer lag time representing a thicker cortex. Input of the estimated cortical thickness, age, height, and weight with proprietary software generates a Density Index (DI), a value that is correlated with BMD at the hip.[35] When DI is substituted for femoral neck BMD in the FRAX algorithm, fracture risk prediction is similar.[35] The findings in several studies suggest the PEUS measurements at the proximal tibia have potential clinical utility for identifying postmenopausal women likely to have or not have osteoporosis, and therefore might be used to identify those who could benefit from further testing by DXA.[36–38] When DXA is not available, DI derived from PEUS could be used with the FRAX algorithm to estimate fracture risk.

IMAGING FOR VERTEBRAL FRACTURES

Vertebral fractures are the most common type of osteoporotic fracture, although most patients with vertebral fractures are not aware of their presence. Conversely, many patients who believe they have had a vertebral fracture do not have one when spine imaging is performed. In an analysis of 1330 men and women in the US National Health and Nutrition Examination Survey (NHANES), only 8% of individuals with a vertebral fracture on imaging had a self-reported fracture, and of those with a self-reported vertebral fracture, only 21% were found to have a vertebral fracture with imaging.[39]

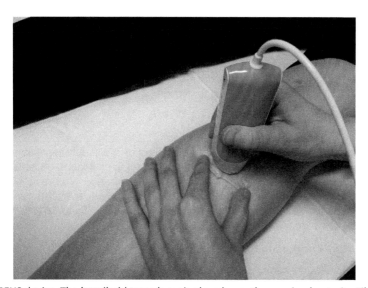

Fig. 1. PEUS device. The handheld transducer is placed over the proximal anterior tibia after application of ultrasound gel to the measurement area. Cortical thickness is estimated by measuring the lag time between ultrasound echoes from the front and back surfaces of the cortex. The signals are transmitted to the connected computer, which then provides a calculated value for DI that is correlated with hip BMD. (*Courtesy of* Janne Karjalainen, PhD, Kuopio, FI.)

Having a vertebral fracture increases the risk of future fractures, with the risk directly correlated with the number of fractures, the severity of the fractures, and the recency of the fractures.[40] Identification of previously unrecognized vertebral fractures may change diagnostic classification from normal or osteopenia to osteoporosis, alter assessment of fracture risk, and influence treatment decisions.[5] Knowledge of a vertebral fracture, especially a recent one, could lead to a decision to start pharmacologic therapy or to select more aggressive therapy than what might otherwise have been used. Indications for spine imaging to detect vertebral fractures have been established by organizations such as the ISCD.[41] The following methods for diagnosing vertebral fractures can be helpful in managing patients in clinical practice.

Vertebral Fracture Assessment

VFA is lateral imaging of the spine by DXA for the purpose of diagnosing vertebral fractures. It can be done in conjunction with BMD measurement by DXA, with greater patient convenience, less radiation, and lower cost than conventional spine radiography. VFA also provides a rapid scan time for the thoracic and lumbar spine without the distortion from parallax and magnification of the image than can occur with standard radiography. VFA is clinically useful for diagnosing grade 2 and grade 3 fractures (Genant semiquantitative technique)[42] at vertebral levels T7 through L4.[43] It performs less well at visualizing levels T4 to T6 compared with conventional radiography, probably because of differences in image resolution and the confounding effects of overlying tissue; however, this is not a great clinical problem, because osteoporosis fractures do not commonly occur at these levels.[44] In a prospective randomized controlled study of 1084 ambulatory elderly women (mean age 75 years), those with vertebral fractures identified by VFA at baseline had up to a 3.8 times increased risk for incident fractures over a follow-up period of 14.5 years.[45] An analysis of 9972 men and women in the Manitoba Bone Density database also showed a robust correlation between vertebral fracture identified by VFA and the risk of future fractures, demonstrating for the first time that imaging of the spine outside the research setting can predict fracture risk.[46] The strength of the association between a prevalent vertebral fracture and subsequent fractures was similar with VFA in these studies and conventional spine X-rays in other large observational cohort studies. Modest training of nonradiologist interpreters of VFA has been shown to provide a high level of accuracy of results compared with radiologists.[47]

Spine Radiography

Spine radiographs have been the traditional method of choice for identifying vertebral fractures in clinical trials and are still commonly used in clinical practice. Compared with VFA, image resolution is better, with better visualization of cortical edges and vertebral endplates. However, upgrades of DXA equipment over the past decade have improved resolution, with better visualization of levels T4 to T6 and high level of accuracy compared with conventional radiographs.[48]

Opportunistic Identification of Vertebral Fractures

There is considerable evidence that vertebral fractures are underreported by radiologists.[49–51] When radiographs, CT scans, MRI studies, and radionuclide scans are performed for a wide variety of indications, vertebral fractures may be identifiable on the images but not mentioned in the report.[52] This highlights the importance of educating interpreters of these studies to recognize and report vertebral fractures, and provides opportunities to use automated computer-aided tools to analyze the images in real-time or review archived images to diagnose vertebral fractures. DXA images with

BMD testing, without VFA, may also incidentally reveal deformities consistent with vertebral fractures. Collectively, these methods constitute opportunistic (fortuitous) identification of vertebral fractures (**Fig. 2**). Opportunistic diagnosis is cost-effective and can improve patient care when high-risk patients are recognized and treatment to reduce fracture risk is initiated.[52]

FRACTURE RISK ALGORITHMS

Because bone strength and fracture risk are determined by more than BMD alone, fracture risk prediction tools have been developed to assist with making clinical decisions. Online fracture risk assessment tools with robust supporting data include FRAX,[20,31] the Garvan Fracture Risk Calculator (Garvan),[53,54] and QFracture.[55,56] FRAX, the tool that is mostly widely used internationally, estimates the 10-year probability of major osteoporotic fracture (hip, forearm, spine, and shoulder) and hip fracture based on input of clinical risk factors for fracture, femoral neck BMD, when available, and TBS, when available. Garvan output is the incidence of any fragility fracture (ie, all fractures excluding digits) and hip fracture over 5 and 10 years, with input of fewer risk factors than FRAX but inclusion of the number of prior fractures and number of falls in the past 12 months, both of which are not part of FRAX. QFracture, used in the United Kingdom, estimates the incidence of hip, wrist, shoulder, or spine fracture and hip fracture over a time period of any number of years from 1 to 10, with input of

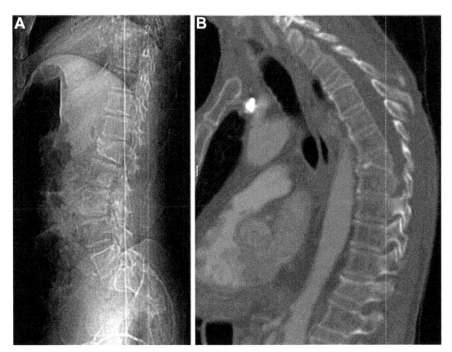

Fig. 2. Opportunistic CT for diagnosing vertebral fractures. CT scans of the chest or abdomen performed for nonskeletal indications can be used to fortuitously diagnosis vertebral fractures without the need for additional scanning or exposure to ionizing radiation. (*A*) Lateral scout image preceding a CT study shows a grade 2 fracture of the upper endplate of L1. (*B*) Midline sagittal reformation of a multidetector CT scan in a different patient shows grade 3 fractures at T3 and T7. (*From* Adams JE. Opportunistic Identification of Vertebral Fractures. J Clin Densitom. 2016;19(1):54-62; with permission.)

many more clinical risk factors than FRAX or Garvan, without the option of including a BMD measurement.

MEASUREMENTS OF BONE STRUCTURE
Bone Geometry

Non-BMD measurements derived from DXA include hip axis length (HAL), the distance from the inner pelvic brim to the greater trochanter.[57] The ISCD has determined that longer HAL is associated with greater hip fracture risk in postmenopausal women, and that other hip geometry parameters (eg, cross-sectional area, cross-sectional moment of inertia, neck shaft angle) should not be used to assess hip fracture risk.[58] An analysis of the Manitoba Bone Density Database found a relative increase in hip fracture probability of 4.7% for every millimeter that HAL is above the sex-specific average for both men and women.[59] This risk is independent of BMD and FRAX probability. The clinical application of HAL measurements is limited due to insufficient reference data in many populations. Hip geometry measurement should not be used to initiate treatment or for monitoring.

Trabecular Bone Score

TBS (TBS iNsight software; Medimaps Group, Geneva, Switzerland) is a textural index that evaluates pixel gray-level variations of the DXA lumbar spine image (**Fig. 3**). TBS provides an indirect assessment of trabecular microarchitecture[60,61] that is

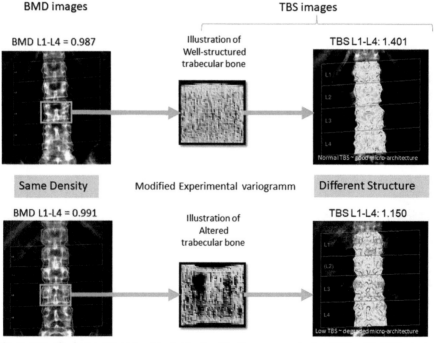

Fig. 3. TBS. The bone strength of individuals with the same or similar BMD with DXA can be different when bone structure is different. TBS measures pixel gray-level variations derived from lumbar spine DXA data. This provides an indirect assessment of trabecular microarchitecture that predicts fracture risk independently of BMD. (*Courtesy of* Didier Hans, PhD, Lausanne, CH.)

independent of BMD.[62] TBS is associated with vertebral, hip, and major osteoporotic fracture risk in postmenopausal women and with hip fracture risk in men older than 50 years.[63] TBS can be used for input with FRAX and may influence treatment decisions by altering the estimated 10-year fracture probability. It is cleared by the US Food and Drug Administration (FDA) to complement BMD measurements by DXA analysis and clinical assessments of fracture risk.[64] TBS is potentially useful for monitoring the skeletal effects of anabolic therapy,[65] although its role in monitoring antiresorptive therapy is unclear.

High-Resolution Peripheral Quantitative Computed Tomography

The first high-resolution peripheral QCT (HR-pQCT) imaging system was introduced in 2004 (Scanco Medical AG, Brüttiselen, Switzerland). This system (XtremeCT) provided 3-D imaging of cortical and trabecular compartments of the distal radius and distal tibia with a spatial resolution (isotropic voxel dimension) of 82 μm. Bone geometry, microarchitecture, and vBMD could be measured in vivo with a radiation dose less than CT that involves more radiosensitive organs. XtremeCT, which is no longer being manufactured but is available as refurbished systems, has been replaced by XtremeCT II, which has a larger field-of-view and spatial resolution that is improved to 61 μm. There is evidence that HR-pQCT can predict fracture risk as well as or better than DXA.[66–68] HR-pQCT (**Fig. 4**) is not currently approved for clinical use; however, it has provided helpful insights into the nature of skeletal disorders in which fracture risk is out of proportion to BMD measured by DXA. As an example, type 2 diabetes mellitus is associated with an increase of fracture risk despite BMD that is typically normal or better than normal. There is evidence of an increase in cortical porosity by HR-pQCT in patients with type 2 diabetes who have fractured, suggesting that this defect in bone quality may play a role in increasing fracture risk independently of BMD.[69] Primary hyperparathyroidism is a disease that is, associated with high fracture risk at many skeletal sites, despite preferential bone loss at the one-third radius, a skeletal site that is mostly cortical bone, and relative preservation of BMD at skeletal sites with a larger proportional of trabecular bone. Studies with HR-pQCT have shown net loss of trabecular bone as well as cortical bone that is, not fully captured by DXA BMD.[70,71] This may explain, at least in part, why fracture risk in these patients is increased at "trabecular" skeletal sites, such as the spine.

High-Resolution MRI

MRI is an attractive technology for 3-D imaging of bone at peripheral (eg, calcaneus, tibia, distal radius) and central (eg, proximal femur) skeletal sites without the use of ionizing radiation. In vitro studies have shown that measurements of trabecular bone structure with high-resolution MRI (HR-MRI) are correlated with bone strength.[72] Limitations include spatial resolution that is above the range for cortical and trabecular microstructure, long scan times, and claustrophobia for some patients.[73] Further advances in HR-MRI technology and correlation with fracture risk are needed before it can be considered useful for clinical applications.

Biomechanical Computed Tomography

Biomechanical CT (BCT) refers to the use of data from CT scans for finite element analysis (FEA) and calculation of DXA-equivalent T-scores at the hip.[74,75] FEA is a general purpose mathematical modeling technique to evaluate the behavior of structures subjected to external loads. This method of structural analysis has been applied to many aspects of engineering since the 1950s, and is especially useful in assessing the strength of loaded structures with complex geometric shapes, including bones such

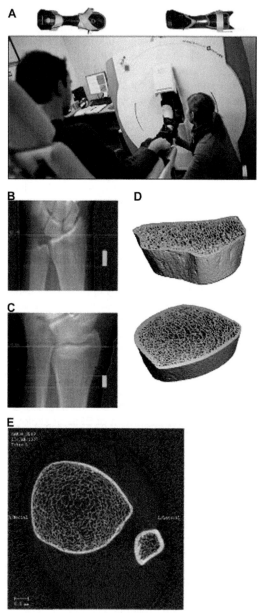

Fig. 4. HR-pQCT. (*A*) Casts used for securing the forearm and lower leg are shown above a photograph of a patient being prepared for measurement of the lower leg. (*B, C, D*) Scout view images of the radius or tibia (*left*) are obtained before selecting the region of interest for the 3-D scan (*right*). (*E*) This is a typical section for HR-pQCT of the ultradistal tibia and fibula. (*From* Cheung AM, Adachi JD, Hanley DA, Kendler DL, Davison KS, Josse R, et al. High-resolution peripheral quantitative computed tomography for the assessment of bone strength and structure: a review by the Canadian Bone Strength Working Group. Curr Osteoporos Rep. 2013;11(2):136-46; with permission.)

as the proximal femur and vertebral bodies. With BCT, 3-D images of hip and spine are divided into smaller elements in a process called "meshing." Material properties are assigned to each element based on gray-scale information from the CT scan that is usually derived from cadaver experiments. Finally, a loading scenario (eg, a sideways fall with a force applied to the greater trochanter of the hip) is simulated using computer software (**Fig. 5**). The main outcome parameter is an estimate of whole-bone strength expressed as newtons (N), the amount of force necessary for a virtual fracture to occur. This integrates factors that include 3-D bone geometry and spatial distribution of cortical and trabecular bone density. Bone strength is then classified as fragile, low, or normal. BCT estimates of bone strength at the spine and hip have been validated in cadaver studies showing that BCT is superior to other commonly used methods, such DXA and QCT.[76,77] VirtuOst (ON Diagnostics, Berkley, CA) is currently the only FDA-cleared BCT software; it is indicated to assess fracture risk, identify

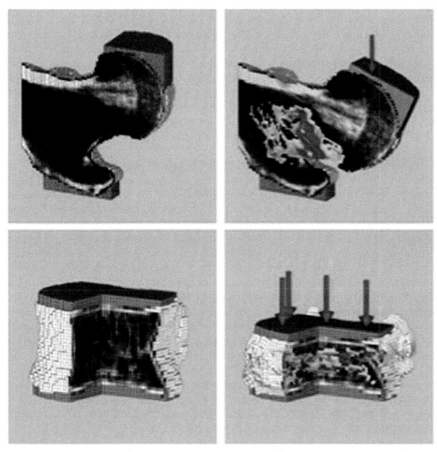

Fig. 5. BCT. Data derived from CT are used to generated finite elements models of the hip (*top*) and spine (*bottom*), sectioned to show internal detail before virtual loading (*left*) and the deformed shape after virtual loading (*right*). The amount of force necessary to deform (fracture) the bone is correlated with bone strength and the risk of fractures. (*From* Keaveny TM, Clarke BL, Cosman F, et al. Biomechanical Computed Tomography analysis (BCT) for clinical assessment of osteoporosis. Osteoporos Int. 2020;31(6):1025-1048; with permission.)

osteoporosis, and monitor therapy. Skeletal FEA has also been applied to data derived from DXA[78] and MRI studies,[79] potentially expanding the clinical applications of this technology.

Limitations of BCT include the inconvenience and expense of having a CT scan, with exposure to ionizing radiation that is much greater than DXA. However, these limitations are overcome when BCT is done opportunistically on CT scans performed for other indications, thereby exposing the patient to no additional radiation or inconvenience.

The ISCD Official Positions state that QCT-based FEA can be used to (1) predict vertebral fracture and hip fractures in postmenopausal women and older men, (2) initiate pharmacologic therapy using validated thresholds in conjunction with clinical risk factors, and (3) monitor age-related and treatment-related changes.[80]

REFERENCE POINT INDENTATION

Microindentation testing is a method for measuring the hardness of a material (eg, metals, ceramics) on a microscopic scale, with hardness often defined as resistance to penetration or permanent deformation with an applied load of known force. The same principles have been applied to in vivo measurement of bone mechanical properties in humans with reference point indentation (RPI). Two devices, using different RPI techniques, have been developed. BioDent (Active Life Scientific, Inc., Santa Barbara, CA) is a device that is usually mounted, used primarily in preclinical research studies with a technique of cyclic RPI (cRPI).[81] OsteoProbe (Active Life Scientific, Inc., Santa Barbara, CA) is a handheld device (**Fig. 6**) for clinical use with impact RPI (iRPI).[82] With both devices, a probe is placed on the surface of a weight-bearing bone (eg, anterior tibia), a force is applied, and the depth of penetration in the outer bone cortex is measured. With cRPI, repeated indentations (up to 20) are made with a force of 2 to 10 N over several seconds, typically repeated 3 to 5 times at nearby bone. The "reference point" is established by the position of the reference probe on the bone surface, with the indentations made by an inner test probe. The outputs most often reported are the total indent distance and the difference between the first ident and the last indent, averaged for the number of tests performed, expressed as microns. With iRPI, a single indentation is made with a greater force (40 N) over a shorter time (0.25 ms), and usually repeated 5 to 10 times in adjacent bone. The reference point is the position of the probe after an initial force of 10 N is applied. The output of iRPI is bone material strength index (BMSI), a dimensionless ratio of averaged indent distances in bone and a reference material composed of polymethylmethacrylate. Although there are similarities with cRPI and iRPI, the differences are great enough that the results cannot be compared; it is likely that different properties of bone tissue are being measured.[83] A notable limitation of both methods is that only the outer cortex (100–200 μm) of bone is measured, with uncertainty as to how well that assesses the material properties of the entire cortex at skeletal sites of major fracture concern, such as the proximal femur and spine. The ultimate clinical utility of iRPI lies in its potential ability to predict fractures, which must be ascertained by sufficiently powered prospective clinical trials which are yet to be done.

FUTURE PERSPECTIVES

DXA is well-established as the gold-standard technology for assessing skeletal health with clinical research and in clinical practice; it is likely to remain so in the foreseeable future. DXA T-scores are typically used to select individuals for participation in clinical trials that have led to regulatory approval of medications to treat patients with

A 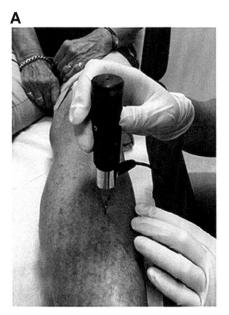   **B**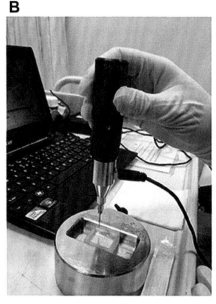

Fig. 6. Impact microindentation. (*A*) The OsteoProbe microindentation device is placed on the midshaft of the anterior tibia after application of a local anesthetic. (*B*) The same device is calibrated with the polymethylmethacrylate reference phantom. (*From* Schoeb M, Hamdy NAT, Malgo F, Winter EM, Appelman-Dijkstra NM. Added Value of Impact Microindentation in the Evaluation of Bone Fragility: A Systematic Review of the Literature. Front Endocrinol (Lausanne). 2020;11:15; with permission.)

osteoporosis. In clinical practice, patients are often started on treatment because of a low DXA T-score. Add-on DXA software, such as TBS and VFA, have enhanced the clinical utility of DXA. Limitations of DXA include cost, availability, use of ionizing radiation, large size and lack of portability for central DXA systems, the need for well-trained technologists and interpreters, and inability to measure all determinants of skeletal strength. None of the other technologies discussed here fully overcomes all of these limitations, but each may address one or more of them.

In locations where DXA availability is limited, ultrasound technologies, such as QUS and PEUS, may be used to screen patients who might benefit from DXA; where there is no availability of DXA, they could be used to identify patients for treatment. Fracture risk algorithms, such as FRAX, with or without BMD input, may also be used to identify patients for treatment. Opportunistic identification of vertebral fractures is currently not widely used, but is very cost-effective and could easily be implemented now. Structural analysis of bone with opportunistic FEA by BCT is available at this time; however, CT performed for the purpose of FEA is likely to remain primarily a research tool. RPI and complex costly technologies, such as HR-pQCT and HR-MRI provide useful information for clinical research but are currently not practical in clinical practice due to cost and availability issues.

SUMMARY

Assessment of bone strength is a critical component in estimating fracture risk and determining which patients are most likely to benefit from pharmacologic therapy to reduce fracture risk. BMD testing with DXA is commonly used in clinical practice to diagnose osteoporosis, assess fracture risk, evaluate bone geometry, and monitor the effects of treatment. Fracture risk algorithms that include clinical risk factors as well as BMD predict fractures better than BMD or clinical risk factors alone. Advanced technologies with 3-D imaging can measure volumetric BMD in cortical and trabecular compartments. High-resolution techniques measure parameters of bone microarchitecture. Mathematical modeling of CT data can be used to estimate resistance to fracture with different types of virtual loading. Minimally invasive techniques can measure bone material properties at the outer cortical surface. Established technologies provide guidance in the management of patients with osteoporosis, and those technologies that are developing and emerging provide insights regarding mechanisms of skeletal fragility and effects of osteoporosis treatments.

CLINICS CARE POINTS

- DXA is the standard method for diagnosing osteoporosis in postmenopausal women and men age 50 years and older.
- VFA and TBS with DXA provide enhanced assessment of fracture risk with the fracture risk algorithm, FRAX.
- Advanced imaging technologies that measure bone microarchitecture and strength have potential clinical applications.

ACKNOWLEDGMENTS

None.

CONFLICTS OF INTEREST

The author has no direct income from potentially conflicting entities. His employer, New Mexico Clinical Research & Osteoporosis Center, has received research grants from Radius, Amgen, Mereo, Bindex; income for service on scientific advisory boards or consulting for Amgen, Radius, Alexion; service on speakers' bureaus for Radius, Alexion; project development for the University of New Mexico; and royalties from UpToDate for sections on DXA, fracture risk assessment, and prevention of osteoporosis. He is a board member of the National Osteoporosis Foundation and the Osteoporosis Foundation of New Mexico.

REFERENCES

1. Kleinert A. Der messende Luchs. NTM 2009;17:199–206.
2. Klibanski A, Adams-Campbell L, Bassford T, et al. Osteoporosis prevention, diagnosis, and therapy. JAMA 2001;285(6):785–95.
3. International Osteoporosis Foundation. Facts and statistics 2020. Available at: https://www.iofbonehealth.org/facts-statistics#category-14. Accessed February 21, 2020.
4. Lewiecki EM. Bone densitometry and vertebral fracture assessment. Curr Osteoporos Rep 2010;8(3):123–30.
5. Lewiecki EM, Laster AJ. Clinical applications of vertebral fracture assessment by dual-energy X-ray absorptiometry. J Clin Endocrinol Metab 2006;91(11):4215–22.
6. Silva BC, Leslie WD, Resch H, et al. Trabecular bone score: a noninvasive analytical method based upon the DXA image. J Bone Miner Res 2014;29(3):518–30.

7. Beck TJ, Broy SB. Measurement of hip geometry-technical background. J Clin Densitom 2015;18(3):331–7.
8. Golestani R, Tio R, Zeebregts CJ, et al. Abdominal aortic calcification detected by dual X-ray absorptiometry: a strong predictor for cardiovascular events. Ann Med 2010;42(7):539–45.
9. Albanese CV, Diessel E, Genant HK. Clinical applications of body composition measurements using DXA. J Clin Densitom 2003;6(2):75–85.
10. Cheng XG, Lowet G, Boonen S, et al. Prediction of vertebral and femoral strength in vitro by bone mineral density measured at different skeletal sites. J Bone Miner Res 1998;13(9):1439–43.
11. Marshall D, Johnell O, Wedel H. Meta-analysis of how well measures of bone mineral density predict occurrence of osteoporotic fractures. BMJ 1996;312(7041):1254–9.
12. Cranney A, Tugwell P, Wells G, et al. Systematic reviews of randomized trials in osteoporosis: Introduction and methodology. Endocr Rev 2002;23(4):497–507.
13. Bouxsein ML, Eastell R, Lui LY, et al. Change in bone density and reduction in fracture risk: a meta-regression of published trials. J Bone Miner Res 2019; 34(4):632–42.
14. Mazess RB, Peppler WW, Harrison JE, et al. Total body bone mineral and lean body mass by dual-photon absorptiometry. III. Comparison with trunk calcium by neutron activation analysis. Calcif Tissue Int 1981;33(4):365–8.
15. Njeh CF, Fuerst T, Hans D, et al. Radiation exposure in bone mineral density assessment. Appl Radiat Isot 1999;50(1):215–36.
16. Bonnick SL. Bone densitometry in clinical practice: application and interpretation. 3rd edition. New York, NY: Humana; 2010.
17. Engelke K, Adams JE, Armbrecht G, et al. Clinical use of quantitative computed tomography and peripheral quantitative computed tomography in the management of osteoporosis in adults: the 2007 ISCD Official Positions. J Clin Densitom 2008;11(1):123–62.
18. Lewiecki EM, Binkley N, Morgan SL, et al. Best practices for dual-energy X-ray absorptiometry measurement and reporting: international society for clinical densitometry guidance. J Clin Densitom 2016;19(2):127–40.
19. Shuhart CR, Yeap SS, Anderson PA, et al. Executive summary of the 2019 ISCD position development conference on monitoring treatment, DXA cross-calibration and least significant change, spinal cord injury, periprosthetic and orthopedic bone health, transgender medicine, and pediatrics. J Clin Densitom 2019; 22(4):453–71.
20. Kanis JA, on behalf of the World Health Organization Scientific Group. Assessment of osteoporosis at the primary health-care level. In: Technical Report. World health organization collaborating centre for metabolic bone diseases, University of Sheffield. UK: Printed by the University of Sheffield; 2007.
21. Morgan SL, Prater GL. Quality in dual-energy X-ray absorptiometry scans. Bone 2017;104:13–28.
22. Curtis JR, Carbone L, Cheng H, et al. Longitudinal trends in use of bone mass measurement among older Americans, 1999-2005. J Bone Miner Res 2008; 23(7):1061–7.
23. Khosla S, Cauley JA, Compston J, et al. Addressing the crisis in the treatment of osteoporosis: a path forward. J Bone Miner Res 2017;32(3):424–30.
24. Lewiecki EM, Chastek B, Sundquist K, et al. Osteoporotic fracture trends in a population of US managed care enrollees from 2007 to 2017. Osteoporos Int 2020;31(7):1299–304.

25. Urrutia J, Besa P, Piza C. Incidental identification of vertebral compression fractures in patients over 60 years old using computed tomography scans showing the entire thoraco-lumbar spine. Arch Orthop Trauma Surg 2019;139(11): 1497–503.

26. Anderson PA, Polly DW, Binkley NC, et al. Clinical use of opportunistic computed tomography screening for osteoporosis. J Bone Joint Surg Am 2018;100(23): 2073–81.

27. Berrington de Gonzalez A, Mahesh M, Kim KP, et al. Projected cancer risks from computed tomographic scans performed in the United States in 2007. Arch Intern Med 2009;169(22):2071–7.

28. Zhang J, Delzell E, Zhao H, et al. Central DXA utilization shifts from office-based to hospital-based settings among Medicare beneficiaries in the wake of reimbursement changes. J Bone Miner Res 2012;27(4):858–64.

29. Troy KL, Edwards WB. Practical considerations for obtaining high quality quantitative computed tomography data of the skeletal system. Bone 2018;110:58–65.

30. American College of Radiology. ACR–SPR–SSR practice parameter for the performance of musculoskeletal quantitative computed tomography (QCT) 2018:1-14. Available at: https://www.acr.org/-/media/ACR/Files/Practice-Parameters/QCT.pdf. Accessed April 5, 2020.

31. University of Sheffield. FRAX fracture risk assessment tool 2020. Available at: http://www.shef.ac.uk/FRAX/. Accessed April 30, 2020.

32. Humbert L, Bague A, Di Gregorio S, et al. DXA-Based 3D analysis of the cortical and trabecular bone of hip fracture postmenopausal women: a case-control study. J Clin Densitom 2020;23(3):403–10.

33. Moayyeri A, Adams JE, Adler RA, et al. Quantitative ultrasound of the heel and fracture risk assessment: an updated meta-analysis. Osteoporos Int 2012; 23(1):143–53.

34. Krieg MA, Barkmann R, Gonnelli S, et al. Quantitative ultrasound in the management of osteoporosis: the 2007 ISCD Official Positions. J Clin Densitom 2008; 11(1):163–87.

35. Karjalainen JP, Riekkinen O, Toyras J, et al. Multi-site bone ultrasound measurements in elderly women with and without previous hip fractures. Osteoporos Int 2012;23(4):1287–95.

36. Karjalainen JP, Riekkinen O, Toyras J, et al. New method for point-of-care osteoporosis screening and diagnostics. Osteoporos Int 2016;27(3):971–7.

37. Schousboe JT, Riekkinen O, Karjalainen J. Prediction of hip osteoporosis by DXA using a novel pulse-echo ultrasound device. Osteoporos Int 2017;28(1):85–93.

38. Karjalainen JP, Riekkinen O, Kroger H. Pulse-echo ultrasound method for detection of post-menopausal women with osteoporotic BMD. Osteoporos Int 2018; 29(5):1193–9.

39. Cosman F, Krege JH, Looker AC, et al. Spine fracture prevalence in a nationally representative sample of US women and men aged >/=40 years: results from the National Health and Nutrition Examination Survey (NHANES) 2013-2014. Osteoporos Int 2017;28(6):1857–66.

40. Ensrud KE, Schousboe JT. Clinical practice. Vertebral fractures. N Engl J Med 2011;364(17):1634–42.

41. Rosen HN, Vokes TJ, Malabanan AO, et al. The Official Positions of the International Society for Clinical Densitometry: vertebral fracture assessment. J Clin Densitom 2013;16(4):482–8.

42. Genant HK, Wu CY, Van Kuijk C, et al. Vertebral fracture assessment using a semiquantitative technique. J Bone Miner Res 1993;8(9):1137–48.

43. Binkley N, Krueger D, Gangnon R, et al. Lateral vertebral assessment: a valuable technique to detect clinically significant vertebral fractures. Osteoporos Int 2005; 16(12):1513–8.

44. Melton LJ III, Kan SH, Frye MA, et al. Epidemiology of vertebral fractures in women. Am J Epidemiol 1989;129:1000–11.

45. Prince RL, Lewis JR, Lim WH, et al. Adding lateral spine imaging for vertebral fractures to densitometric screening: improving ascertainment of patients at high risk of incident osteoporotic fractures. J Bone Miner Res 2019;34(2):282–9.

46. Schousboe JT, Lix LM, Morin SN, et al. Prevalent vertebral fracture on bone density lateral spine (VFA) images in routine clinical practice predict incident fractures. Bone 2019;121:72–9.

47. Aubry-Rozier B, Fabreguet I, Iglesias K, et al. Impact of level of expertise versus the statistical tool on vertebral fracture assessment (VFA) readings in cohort studies. Osteoporos Int 2017;28(2):523–7.

48. Diacinti D, Del Fiacco R, Pisani D, et al. Diagnostic performance of vertebral fracture assessment by the lunar iDXA scanner compared to conventional radiography. Calcif Tissue Int 2012;91(5):335–42.

49. Gehlbach SH, Bigelow C, Heimisdottir M, et al. Recognition of vertebral fracture in a clinical setting. Osteoporos Int 2000;11:577–82.

50. Delmas PD, van de Langerijt L, Watts NB, et al. Underdiagnosis of vertebral fractures is a worldwide problem: the IMPACT study. J Bone Miner Res 2005;20(4): 557–63.

51. Bartalena T, Rinaldi MF, Modolon C, et al. Incidental vertebral compression fractures in imaging studies: lessons not learned by radiologists. World J Radiol 2010;2(10):399–404.

52. Adams JE. Opportunistic identification of vertebral fractures. J Clin Densitom 2016;19(1):54–62.

53. Nguyen ND, Frost SA, Center JR, et al. Development of prognostic nomograms for individualizing 5-year and 10-year fracture risks. Osteoporos Int 2008; 19(10):1431–44.

54. Garvan Institute of Medical Research. Bone fracture risk calculator 2020. Available at: http://www.garvan.org.au/bone-fracture-risk/. Accessed April 30, 2020.

55. Hippisley-Cox J, Coupland C. Derivation and validation of updated QFracture algorithm to predict risk of osteoporotic fracture in primary care in the United Kingdom: prospective open cohort study. BMJ 2012;344:e3427.

56. ClinRisk Ltd. Welcome to the QFracture-2016 risk calculator 2020. Available at: https://qfracture.org/. Accessed May 1, 2020.

57. Faulkner KG, Genant HK, McClung M. Bilateral comparison of femoral bone density and hip axis length from single and fan beam DXA scans. Cacif Tissue Int 1995;56(1):26–31.

58. Broy SB, Cauley JA, Lewiecki EM, et al. Fracture risk prediction by non-BMD DXA measures: the 2015 ISCD Official Positions Part 1: hip geometry. J Clin Densitom 2015;18(3):287–308.

59. Leslie WD, Lix LM, Morin SN, et al. Adjusting hip fracture probability in men and women using hip axis length: the manitoba bone density database. J Clin Densitom 2016;19(3):326–31.

60. Muschitz C, Kocijan R, Haschka J, et al. TBS reflects trabecular microarchitecture in premenopausal women and men with idiopathic osteoporosis and low-traumatic fractures. Bone 2015;79:259–66.

61. Ramalho J, Marques IDB, Hans D, et al. The trabecular bone score: Relationships with trabecular and cortical microarchitecture measured by HR-pQCT and histomorphometry in patients with chronic kidney disease. Bone 2018;116:215–20.

62. Shevroja E, Lamy O, Kohlmeier L, et al. Use of Trabecular Bone Score (TBS) as a complementary approach to dual-energy X-ray absorptiometry (DXA) for fracture risk assessment in clinical practice. J Clin Densitom 2017;20(3):334–45.

63. Silva BC, Broy SB, Boutroy S, et al. Fracture risk prediction by non-BMD DXA measures: the 2015 ISCD Official Positions Part 2: Trabecular Bone Score. J Clin Densitom 2015;18(3):309–30.

64. US Food and Drug Administration. Indications for Use, TBS iNsight 2016. Available at: https://www.accessdata.fda.gov/cdrh_docs/pdf15/K152299.pdf. Accessed February 2, 2019.

65. Krohn K, Schwartz EN, Chung YS, et al. Dual-energy X-ray absorptiometry monitoring with trabecular bone score: 2019 ISCD Official Position. J Clin Densitom 2019;22(4):501–5.

66. Samelson EJ, Broe KE, Xu H, et al. Cortical and trabecular bone microarchitecture as an independent predictor of incident fracture risk in older women and men in the Bone Microarchitecture International Consortium (BoMIC): a prospective study. Lancet Diabetes Endocrinol 2019;7(1):34–43.

67. Sornay-Rendu E, Boutroy S, Duboeuf F, et al. Bone microarchitecture assessed by HR-pQCT as predictor of fracture risk in postmenopausal women: the OFELY Study. J Bone Miner Res 2017;32(6):1243–51.

68. Litwic AE, Westbury LD, Robinson DE, et al. Bone phenotype assessed by HRpQCT and associations with fracture risk in the GLOW study. Calcif Tissue Int 2018;102(1):14–22.

69. Patsch JM, Burghardt AJ, Yap SP, et al. Increased cortical porosity in type 2 diabetic postmenopausal women with fragility fractures. J Bone Miner Res 2013; 28(2):313–24.

70. Hansen S, Beck Jensen JE, Rasmussen L, et al. Effects on bone geometry, density, and microarchitecture in the distal radius but not the tibia in women with primary hyperparathyroidism: a case-control study using HR-pQCT. J Bone Miner Res 2010;25(9):1941–7.

71. Stein EM, Silva BC, Boutroy S, et al. Primary hyperparathyroidism is associated with abnormal cortical and trabecular microstructure and reduced bone stiffness in postmenopausal women. J Bone Miner Res 2013;28(5):1029–40.

72. Link TM, Vieth V, Langenberg R, et al. Structure analysis of high resolution magnetic resonance imaging of the proximal femur: in vitro correlation with biomechanical strength and BMD. Calcif Tissue Int 2003;72(2):156–65.

73. Link TM, Kazakia G. Update on imaging-based measurement of bone mineral density and quality. Curr Rheumatol Rep 2020;22(5):13.

74. Keaveny TM. Biomechanical computed tomography-noninvasive bone strength analysis using clinical computed tomography scans. Ann N Y Acad Sci 2010; 1192:57–65.

75. Keaveny TM, Clarke BL, Cosman F, et al. Biomechanical Computed Tomography analysis (BCT) for clinical assessment of osteoporosis. Osteoporos Int 2020; 31(6):1025–48.

76. Crawford RP, Cann CE, Keaveny TM. Finite element models predict in vitro vertebral body compressive strength better than quantitative computed tomography. Bone 2003;33(4):744–50.

77. Cody DD, Gross GJ, Hou FJ, et al. Femoral strength is better predicted by finite element models than QCT and DXA. J Biomech 1999;32(10):1013–20.

78. Leslie WD, Luo Y, Yang S, et al. Fracture risk indices from DXA-based finite element analysis predict incident fractures independently from FRAX: The Manitoba BMD Registry. J Clin Densitom 2019;22(3):338–45.
79. Rajapakse CS, Chang G. Micro-finite element analysis of the proximal femur on the basis of high-resolution magnetic resonance images. Curr Osteoporos Rep 2018;16(6):657–64.
80. Zysset P, Qin L, Lang T, et al. Clinical use of quantitative computed tomography-based finite element analysis of the hip and spine in the management of osteoporosis in adults: the 2015 ISCD Official Positions-Part II. J Clin Densitom 2015;18(3):359–92.
81. Diez-Perez A, Guerri R, Nogues X, et al. Microindentation for in vivo measurement of bone tissue mechanical properties in humans. J Bone Miner Res 2010;25(8):1877–85.
82. Schoeb M, Hamdy NAT, Malgo F, et al. Added value of impact microindentation in the evaluation of bone fragility: a systematic review of the literature. Front Endocrinol (Lausanne) 2020;11:15.
83. Allen MR, McNerny EM, Organ JM, et al. True gold or pyrite: a review of reference point indentation for assessing bone mechanical properties in vivo. J Bone Miner Res 2015;30(9):1539–50.

Moving?

Make sure your subscription moves with you!

To notify us of your new address, find your **Clinics Account Number** (located on your mailing label above your name), and contact customer service at:

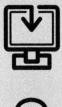

Email: journalscustomerservice-usa@elsevier.com

800-654-2452 (subscribers in the U.S. & Canada)
314-447-8871 (subscribers outside of the U.S. & Canada)

Fax number: 314-447-8029

Elsevier Health Sciences Division
Subscription Customer Service
3251 Riverport Lane
Maryland Heights, MO 63043

Printed and bound by CPI Group (UK) Ltd, Croydon, CR0 4YY

08/05/2025

01864697-0006